PLAY HEALTHY, STAY HEALTHY

Gary N. Guten, MD

Orthopedic Surgeon
Medical Director, Sports Medicine Institute, Milwaukee, WI

Leisure Press
Champaign, Illinois

Library of Congress Cataloging-in-Publication Data

Guten, Gary N., 1939-
   Play healthy, stay healthy / Gary N. Guten.
      p.   cm.
   Includes index.
   ISBN 0-88011-439-8
      1. Sports--Accidents and injuries--Treatment.   2. Athletes-
   -Rehabilitation.   I. Title.
   RD97.G88   1991
   617.1'027--dc20   90-28365
                                                                  CIP

ISBN: 0-88011-439-8

Leisure Press books are available at special discounts for bulk purchase for sales promotions, premiums, fund-raising, or educational use. Special editions or book excerpts can also be created to specification. For details, contact the Special Sales Manager at Leisure Press.

Printed in the United States of America   10   9   8   7   6   5   4   3   2

Leisure Press
A Divison of Human Kinetics
Web site: http:// www.humankinetics.com/

United States: Human Kinetics, P.O. Box 5076, Champaign, IL 61825-5076
1-800-747-4457

Canada: Human Kinetics, Box 24040, Windsor, ON N8Y 4Y9
1-800-465-7301 (in Canada only)

Europe: Human Kinetics, P.O. Box IW14, Leeds LS16 6TR, United Kingdom
(44) 1132 781708

Australia: Human Kinetics, 57A Price Avenue, Lower Mitcham,
South Australia 5062   (08) 277 1555

New Zealand: Human Kinetics, P.O. Box 105-231, Auckland 1
(09) 523 3462

To my patients—by listening to them,
I have learned how to "Play Healthy, Stay Healthy."

To my family—"my pride and joy."

Credits

Acquisitions Editor: Brian Holding
Developmental Editor: Judy Patterson Wright, PhD
Assistant Editors: Julia Anderson and Dawn Levy
Copyeditor: David Severtson
Proofreader: Stefani Day
Indexer: Sheila Ary
Production Director: Ernie Noa
Typesetter: Sandra Meier
Text Design: Keith Blomberg
Text Layout: Tara Welsch
Cover Design: Jack Davis
Interior Art: Janet Sinn and Gretchen Walters
Printer: Versa Press

CONTENTS

Part IV Specific Rehabilitation Exercise Programs 167

PREFACE

This book is written for fitness enthusiasts and athletes who are in training or are injured. It is designed for participants in both team and aerobic sports. The focus is how to handle musculoskeletal injuries by learning to *Play Healthy, Stay Healthy* for guidance in managing sports injuries and answering the "what, why, how, and who" kinds of questions that injured athletes regularly face.

Patients' concerns about their injuries typically center on questions like the following: How much activity can I have? What else can I do? Should I apply heat or cold? What are the appropriate exercises for rehabilitation? What medications should I use? What kind of diet should I be on and what should I drink? What is the best shoe (and other apparel) for my type of exercise? What is the best surface for me to run on? Should I use a brace? The 10-Point Treatment Plan explained in this book evolved in response to such questions.

The signals of a traffic light are used to illustrate three activity levels that can be applied to sports injuries:

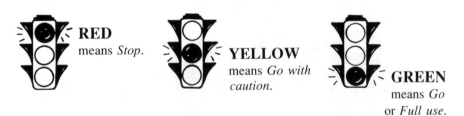

RED means *Stop*.

YELLOW means *Go with caution*.

GREEN means *Go* or *Full use*.

This key is applied to specific injuries and also to different aspects of a treatment plan. The 10-Point Treatment Plan, based on commonly accepted sports medicine practice, is presented in a unique format that is easy to follow and to remember. The plan explains a theory of managing injuries that includes the appropriate activity level for different kinds of injuries.

With this plan, you can learn to listen to your body and establish the best activity level for your injury. My advice is based on the assumption that the most important first step for an injured athlete is to get a correct diagnosis from a health professional. Once you have a correct diagnosis of your problem and a treatment plan, the 10-Point Treatment Plan presented here will put you back on track. Although this plan is relatively new, it emerges from a movement toward physical fitness and self-responsibility that has been evolving during the past 3 decades.

Although people have suffered injuries as a result of physical activity throughout history, it wasn't until the 1960s that exercising was recognized as an essential part of a well-balanced life. Spurred by Dr. Ken Cooper, the world awakened to the concept of aerobic sports—running, biking, and swimming became favorite world-wide activities.

In 1972, we were inspired by the victory of marathon runner Frank Shorter in the Munich Olympics. The explosion of fitness enthusiasts continued. By the late 1970s, the number of runners reached 20 million, with many thousands running marathons. Along with all this activity came an inevitable increase in injuries and the subsequent development of the specialty of "sports medicine."

In the 1980s, athletes embraced the credos of "No pain, no gain" and "Winning is everything." As the intensity of workouts and competition increased, significant injury patterns emerged among fitness enthusiasts. In casual conversation and in the media, we started to hear such phrases as "tennis elbow," "runner's knee," and "rotator cuff." Famous athletes—Frank Shorter, Jim McMahon, Billie Jean King, Joan Benoit, Grete Waitz, Olga Korbut, Mary Decker Slaney, and Sugar Ray Leonard, to name a few—also became famous patients. "Athletic highs" were sometimes replaced by "runner's depression."

Now in the 1990s, the tide is turning. Athletes, fitness enthusiasts, and coaches are awakening to the concepts of listening to your body and letting pain be your guide. In this book, a key word in reference to the newest training and rehabilitation techniques is *moderation*. Derived from the Latin word *moderatus*, moderation means to limit extremes; think of the *moderator* who brings together divergent sides in a discussion. Too much of anything is not good—too much rest is just as bad as too much activity.

The purpose of this sports medicine book is to present a simple treatment plan to help the athlete or person who seriously exercises handle injuries and keep fit for exercising. *Play Healthy, Stay Healthy* provides the injured athlete with a self-help guide for use in conjunction with a physician's or other health professional's treatment plan. This is a unique book about communicating with the professionals (doctors, coaches, and trainers) and about listening to your own body's signals for guidance in taking the necessary steps to recovery. The book is also a resource for the physician or health professional who needs material for patients to use as a guide or for reinforcement of a treatment plan.

Play Healthy, Stay Healthy is organized in a straightforward, easy-to-use format. A standard table of contents outlines the book's topics, but there is also an anatomical contents page illustrating which conditions may affect various body parts and where in the book to turn for advice (see Part III).

Part I discusses responding to your body's signals and answers basic questions: Why should I listen to my body? How should I listen? What people should I listen to? Part II introduces the structure of the rest of the book. After briefly discussing causes and types of injuries, this section describes the Stop, Caution, Go approach to activity levels for different injuries. In general, it explains the 6-Point Condition Summary and describes the 10-Point Treatment Plan that is applied in Part III.

Part III presents 40 Specific Injury Treatments for conditions experienced frequently by athletes. These conditions are organized by body part in roughly a head-to-toe manner. Each condition illustrates the injured body part, lists the specific 6-Point Condition Summary, lists the specific 10-Point Treatment Plan, and indicates the recommended activity level.

Part IV presents the specific rehabilitation exercise programs that are cross-referenced within Part III.

After reading the two introductory sections (Parts I and II), you will understand how the treatment plans work. Then you will be able to listen to your body, find the condition and treatment plan (Part III) for your injury, and follow the recommended rehab exercises (Part IV) while maintaining an appropriate activity level. You will find that your capacity to rebound from an injury and your ability to continue some level of activity will be greatly enhanced by this approach.

Disclaimer: You should note that the medical information and advice in this book is presented only as a guide—it should be used only in conjunction with the advice of your physician or health care provider.

ACKNOWLEDGMENTS

Writing a book is like playing football. The author is the quarterback calling the signals. But it takes an entire team to carry out a winning effort. What follows is a listing of the team members for *Play Healthy, Stay Healthy*.

Developmental Editor	Judy Patterson Wright, PhD
Dietitian	Margaret Klink, RD Director of Food and Nutrition Services
Hospital Librarian	Ann Towell, MA Health Sciences Librarian
Lawyer/Running Companion	Leonard Zubrensky, JD
Management Consultant	Melvin L. Schultz, CPBC Professional Management of Milwaukee
Medical Assistants	Jean Julson and Debbie Miller
Medical Illustrator	Janet Sinn
Office Manager	Kathleen Swosinski
Physician Therapy Supervisor	Debbie Buntrock, PT
Physicians	Harvey Kohn, MD, Orthopedic Surgeon, Donald Zoltan, MD, Orthopedic Surgeon, and Thomas Pietrocarlo, DPM, Podiatrist, Sports Medicine and Knee Surgery Center
Physician Coordinator	Linda Ribbeck
Rehabilitation Director	Tess Maier, RN
Transcriptionist	Clare Bowe, assisted by Gail Mackay and Shelly LaPedus
Writing Associate	Sue Montgomery Montgomery Media, Inc.

The root of the word *acknowledgment* is "knowledge." The people listed here contributed not only hard work and effort but, more important, their knowledge. For this I am very appreciative.

SPECIAL ACKNOWLEDGMENTS

To the Sports Medicine Institute personnel,
Sinai Samaritan Medical Center,
Milwaukee, Wisconsin,
for their help with the rehabilitation exercises
and diet plan presented in this book.

To my office personnel,
Sports Medicine and Knee Surgery Center,
Milwaukee, Wisconsin,
for their patience and dedication.

PART I

● LISTEN
TO YOUR BODY

Too much activity can be as detrimental as too little. Part I explores not only the rewards of regular exercise but also the potential risks associated with certain activities. You can learn to balance and moderate your exercise needs. The answer is simple—listen to your body. Whenever joint and muscle problems develop, your body communicates with you through such symptoms as pain, swelling, stiffness, noise, and instability. These symptoms can come from many sources and should signal you that irritation and injury are occurring.

The following questions are answered in Part I:

- Why is it important to listen to your body?
- How does your body communicate with you?
- Who can you turn to for professional help?
- What can you expect to receive from your physician or health care provider?
- What information can you bring to your health care provider?

Why Listen to Your Body?

Athletes around the world who have experienced a sports injury immediately look outside themselves for a solution to their concerns, but their first step should really be looking and listening to their own bodies. Your body is talking to you—are you listening? Your body is telling you that there are wonderful rewards and some risks when you exercise regularly. By learning how to interpret your body's signals you can work with your health care provider to design a treatment program that will respond precisely to your body's needs.

Participating in sports is similar to investing money. You can put your money in a savings account that pays 5 percent, receive little reward, and have low risk.

Or you can purchase volatile options in the futures market, which can pay tremendous sums, but you risk losing all your money. Somewhere in between, the cautious investor buys prudent stocks and bonds for long-term growth and stability.

Most of us seem to understand the concept of money management but have trouble understanding ''body management'' when it comes to choosing activities. The risks of poor money management are sometimes very clear—bankruptcy, poverty, extreme loss. We sometimes forget the risks of poor body management. We rarely think about the possibility of pain and disability that may accompany sports injuries unless an injury happens to us.

Reward/Risk Ratio

Although you are involved in sports activity because you know some of the potential rewards, occasionally reminding yourself of these rewards may keep you motivated. The rewards of physical activity are many:

- Prevention of musculoskeletal injuries by maintaining muscle tone
- Improved flexibility and range of motion
- Prolonged physical and mental health
- Improved cardiovascular endurance
- Improved positive feeling of ''good health''
- Opportunity to learn new skills
- Opportunities for friendship and socialization
- The fun of games
- Team membership
- For a few, a career, an opportunity to earn ''big money''

This list can go on, but it helps explain why sports are such an important part of our culture. Yet we sometimes lose sight of the fact that millions of people become injured and that some injuries lead to complications, even though most injuries are minor. Some of the specific complications that may result are minor musculoskeletal injury followed by a brief period of disability; major bone and joint injury, which may lead to chronic pain or arthritis; financial losses because of time spent recuperating and because of medical expenses; and mental depression, which occasionally may become severe.

You, the athlete, must decide whether the rewards of your particular sports activity outweigh the potential risks. Younger athletes sometimes have a hard time with balancing rewards and risks because they tend to focus on the rewards and deny the risks. Many teenagers ''live for today,'' which is why pregnancy, AIDS, smoking, and drugs can become such problems. Teenagers frequently deny the risks inherent in dangerous behaviors, but they can also deny the risks involved in positive behaviors such as sports activity. Because of their experience, older athletes are more aware of risks and approach the rewards more realistically.

Complications develop with the extremes. Too much activity may result in injuries leading to some of the problems mentioned earlier, while inactivity can lead to

- weight gain,
- loss of muscle mass,
- loss of bone strength (particularly in women who are prone to developing osteoporosis),
- mental inactivity leading to depression, and
- loss of cardiovascular conditioning.

Mature judgment can lead to the appropriate level of activity.

It is no surprise that young athletes in particular are confused by these potential risks and rewards associated with too much or too little activity. Achieving balance is the goal, but how? The answer is simple—listen to your body.

Our bodies have evolved with a wonderful mechanism for letting us know when we are experiencing too much activity. In a word, the concept is "pain." If you are experiencing increasing aches and discomfort in a muscle or joint, your body is telling you to moderate, reduce activities, rest a while, and change your activity. The worst thing you can do is ignore the pain. This will only aggravate the problem and cause increasing difficulty with healing. How to deal with this pain will be explained more in Part II.

Why Exercise?

Athletes should realize that every activity has a reward/risk ratio. Generally in life, the greater the reward, the greater the risk. A key step for every athlete is to realize why we exercise. Younger athletes generally focus on the competitive aspects of sports activity—specifically on winning. Winning is part of international competition. The famous football coach Vince Lombardi said, "Winning is not everything—it is the only thing!" This quotation generally reflects the viewpoint of the professional athlete. At the professional sports level, with billions of dollars at risk, winning is certainly everything. This emphasis on winning is transmitted to most athletes, even those not involved in professional competition, and can eventually lead to musculoskeletal injuries.

Unless you are a professional athlete, you may discover more benefits in exercising if you focus on factors other than winning, factors such as having fun and becoming physically fit. You will also find sports activity more satisfying if you are continually aware of the potential for injury. It is amazing how cautious you will become after you have experienced your first sports injury. Once you learn to listen to your body and become aware of the signals your body gives, you will be able to avoid many potentially serious injuries and successfully manage injuries once they occur.

How to Listen to Your Body

Being in tune with how your body is reacting to activity is important to all athletes. Just as with most new activities, learning how to listen to your body takes experience and practice; however, once you learn how to understand what your body is telling you, it becomes easier all the time. After all, no one knows your body better than you do.

Your body communicates with you in various ways when joint and muscle problems develop. Pain, swelling, stiffness, noise, and instability are the most common ways your body tells you that something is wrong. Let's look at these symptoms in more detail so you will be aware of them when they occur.

Pain

Think of pain as simply your body's way of telling you (signaling) that injury and irritation are occurring. Pain can come from many sources. It may be due to a buildup of chemicals (such as lactic acid) to stimulate certain nerve fibers in the muscles. Pain may be due to a mechanical cause such as general wear and tear on the body, or it can be caused by inflammation or irritation of the lining of a joint. Whatever the cause, there are basically three types of pain—vague, localized, and delayed. These types are explained more fully in Part II under "Activity Levels" (point 1 of the 10-Point Treatment Plan).

Swelling

Swelling is the accumulation of fluid around or inside a joint or muscle. This is the body's initial way of healing and is also known as the "inflammatory process." The body is trying to bring blood products and fluid to fight the injury and cleanse the injured area. Sometimes the swelling and the inflammatory process cause more problems than the initial injury; however, keep in mind that some swelling is necessary for healing to take place. For practical purposes, consider that a little swelling might be fine, while too much is not good and should be suppressed with anti-inflammatory treatment. Ways to treat swelling will be discussed in the 10-Point Treatment Plan section.

Stiffness

Stiffness can come from inside a joint and can be due to swelling, a torn cartilage, or arthritic spurs in an internal joint. Stiffness can also be caused by factors outside the joint; inflamed or tight muscles or tendons are frequent sources of such stiffness. Generally, stiffness without local pain in the joint is probably a result of muscle injury or muscle inflammation and does not imply a serious problem. Stiffness associated with local pain, though, implies a more serious condition.

Noise

Noises or snaps in the joint can be very confusing. Listening to noises and interpreting them correctly is very important. If the noise or snap is associated with local pain, this generally indicates a potential problem. Noise can be caused by a roughness of the joint surfaces known as chondromalacia or by an irritation of the joint associated with osteoarthritis or torn meniscus; however, in the hip or ankle, the noise can be produced by the simple movement of a normal tendon gliding over a normal bony protrusion and causing a snap.

As a rule of thumb, you should moderate those activities that cause a joint to snap. Even if there is no initial pain, persistent snapping and irritation can lead to roughness and eventual tendinitis. If the joint produces a noise but no pain, stiffness, or swelling, then the noise can generally be monitored without any major change in activity; moderation should be the key.

Instability

Joints are held together with muscles and ligaments. Some joints, such as the shoulders or the knees, are inherently unstable. Other joints, such as the hips, are much more stable. Joint instability or "giving way" can be the result of two different problems. One involves the internal knee joint or ligaments inside or around the knee, for example, the anterior cruciate ligament. The other problem may involve factors in the muscles around the joint—for example, a weak thigh, which causes the knee to give way.

Giving way and instability can be serious problems and should not be ignored. Giving way, even without pain, should be carefully assessed by a health care provider. At first, instability should be treated by simply restricting those activities that cause it, working on building muscles around the joint, and carefully evaluating and treating the joint factors, such as a torn ligament or a loose body within the joint.

Whom to Listen to

As much as you need to be responsible for your own well-being, you also need to be able to work with health professionals who have the experience and knowledge to guide you in the right direction. There are many health care providers who can help you, including physicians and other professionals who practice the relatively new specialty of sports medicine. With so many specialists and so much help available, the injured athlete and consumer can be very confused. When you are injured, who should you contact for help?

Sources of Help

The chart below lists various health professionals and other providers of help and their special expertise and skills.

Health Care Provider	Definition
Medical doctors	MDs, or physicians who practice family medicine, internal medicine, general surgery, and orthopedic surgery. They are trained in medical diagnosis and treatment.
Orthopedic surgeons	MDs who are trained specifically in injuries of the musculoskeletal system; team physicians of most major sports are orthopedic surgeons. "Ortho" means straight (not bones) and "pedic" means child (not foot). Orthopedic surgeons of the 18th and 19th centuries treated the musculoskeletal deformities of growing children. Now they treat injuries in athletes.
Osteopaths	DOs, or doctors of osteopathy. "Osteo" refers to bone. Osteopaths' philosophy of medicine is based on the theory that the body is capable of making its own remedies against disease when it is in a normal structural relationship. Chief emphasis is on the importance of normal body mechanics and manipulative methods.
Podiatrists	DPMs, or doctors of podiatric medicine, who specialize in care of the foot and associated injuries. Highly specialized surgical procedures are done in conjunction with orthopedic surgeons.
Chiropractors	DCs, or doctors of chiropractic medicine, which is based on the theory that health and disease are related to the function of the nervous system. Diagnosis is done by identifying the irritants, and treatment is done by conservative manipulative and massage techniques. Some athletes find chiropractors very helpful in treating muscular injuries, though it is very unusual for a chiropractor to be the primary team physician for a high school, college, or professional team.

Nurses	RNs, or registered nurses; health care providers who work in close conjunction with physicians and hospitals to rehabilitate and treat injured athletes. You might not initially go directly to a nurse for an injury, but a nurse may be one of your primary caregivers.
Physical therapists	PTs; allied health professionals who deal with the diagnosis, treatment, and prevention of disease with the aid of physical agents such as light, heat, cold, water, and mechanical apparatus for musculoskeletal rehabilitation. Physical therapists work in close conjunction with physicians and orthopedic surgeons for treatment and rehabilitation. In a few select states, physical therapists are allowed to make a diagnosis and render treatment without a physician's prescription.
Trainers	ATCs, or certified athletic trainers; health professionals trained to diagnose and provide first aid on the practice field. They provide specialized instruction, training techniques, instruction in prevention of injuries, and immediate first aid. They work in close conjunction with physical therapists and physicians.
Coaches	The "health educators" most involved in training and rehabilitation of the athlete. At times, the coach is the first person to see the injured athlete, and coaches sometimes give advice on the management of pain.
Teachers	Frequent advisers on exercise physiology, nutrition, biology, and sports. Like coaches, teachers may walk a fine line between teaching and managing minor injuries.
Parents	Potential caretakers in educating and rendering first aid to an injured child. They can have a tremendous positive effect on guiding young athletes.
Friends	Persons often turned to for advice. Friends can be helpful in providing encouragement and in guiding you to a reliable health care provider; however, they can be the least reliable source of medical information.
You	At times the best "health provider"—especially if you have learned the principles in this book and are able to listen to your body. Only you can fully understand your own pain level. If you learn to modify activities according to pain levels, you can be of great help to yourself in managing an injury. The 10-Point Treatment Plan

outlined in this book can help you in conjunction with your doctor's diagnosis and treatment recommendations.

Obviously, there are so many possible sources of information that it can be very confusing to know where to turn for help. Who do you turn to for advice? There are many key considerations—cost, time, and the effect on your social life and activity level. You may use this list as a guideline in sorting out alternatives for help; however, one of the best approaches is choosing a health care provider based on a reference from a friend who has had a similar problem and has been treated successfully. Here are some other resources for finding a good health care provider:

- Call the Medical Society of your community. Ask for a sports medicine specialist—generally an orthopedic surgeon.
- Call the local college health department and ask for their sports medicine specialist.
- Call the American Orthopaedic Society for Sports Medicine in Chicago at (312) 644-2623 for a national directory of community listings of orthopedic surgeons who specialize in sports medicine.
- Call a local hospital and ask for a referral to an orthopedic surgeon specializing in sports medicine.
- Call one of the national computerized physician referral services.

A sports injury can be a prolonged, frustrating problem. Your first step is to listen to your body and then seek help. If your health care provider simply says, "stop all activity, go home, and do nothing," then you may want to seek a second opinion. Keep in mind that the 10-Point Treatment Plan explained later in this book is designed to help you in conjunction with your doctor's advice.

Working With Your Physician

Finding the right physician or health care provider to help you handle your injury is the first step. The next step is working well with that person so that the best results can be achieved. It is important to know how your physician organizes information and what kinds of help to expect.

If you understand how your doctor organizes records, you can help organize your thoughts, and your injury management will be much more effective. You will find that most physicians use a chart to organize your medical problems into four components: Subjective, Objective, Assessment, and Plan. Your doctor probably calls this the SOAP method. These important components are described here.

Subjective

This is the history that you give the physician and includes the symptoms you perceive, for example, pain, stiffness, swelling, throbbing, or numbness. In medical school, students are taught that the history forms 85 percent of the diagnosis and is the most important aspect of the diagnosis. If you write down and organize these concerns before you see the doctor, you will save time and help your physician (see Figure 1.1).

Injury Form

1. **Where** does your pain seem to be located?
2. **What** are the symptoms?
   - Pain?
   - Swelling?
   - Stiffness?
   - Instability?
3. **When** did these symptoms begin?
4. What (do you believe) **caused** this injury?
5. What activity or movement **increases** your pain or other symptoms?
6. What, if anything, have you been doing to **treat** this injury?
7. **Past** medical history, including dates, injuries, and previous treatments.
8. **Medication** now being taken?
9. Any **allergy** to medication?
10. **Who** referred you to the doctor (so a report can be sent)?

Figure 1.1   Form for patient to fill out before seeing doctor.

Objective

This is what physicians perceive with their senses of sight, hearing, and touch. The physician may detect a lump, muscle atrophy, soft tissue swelling, local tenderness, or joint instability. These are all objective findings that aid in the diagnosis. Other possible objective findings come from X-rays, MRI tests, and arthrograms.

Assessment

This is the diagnosis—the physician's conclusion of what is wrong with you. An accurate assessment is derived when the physician puts together your subjective and objective findings. This is the most important reason you seek medical care—to obtain a proper diagnosis. The physician will explain to you how this diagnosis was reached.

Plan

This is the treatment program for your specific diagnosis. Part II of this book explains how an effective 10-Point Treatment Plan is organized, and Part III looks at specific treatment plans for 40 common injuries.

When you consult a health care provider, you should seek an understanding of three key components: a diagnosis, options, and complications. You can remember these three words with the acronym DOC. You are probably most interested in a proper diagnosis, but you should make sure you understand your options and the possible complications of each treatment plan. If you were a patient in our office, we would advise you that ultimately you make the final decision about treatment, based on your understanding of the three key components. When you understand them, you will be able to apply a specific 10-Point Treatment Plan.

HOW TO TREAT
AN INJURY

Part II (a) identifies how you can reduce your chances of injury; (b) explains the types of injuries; (c) introduces you to the Stop, Caution, Go approach to treating injuries; (d) details the 6-Point Condition Summary for proper diagnosis; and (e) presents the 10-Point Treatment Plan, which represents the 10 most frequent physician recommendations.

Each condition summary includes these six points:

1. Definition
2. Cause
3. Subjective symptoms
4. Objective findings
5. Testing procedures
6. Prognosis

Each treatment plan looks at 10 key aspects of treating an injury:

1. Activity levels
2. Alternative activities
3. Rehab exercises
4. Support
5. Thermal treatment
6. Medication
7. Equipment
8. Nutrition
9. Fluids
10. Surfaces

In particular, the activity level category will guide you toward the right amount of activity based on which one of three types of pain you might have: vague, localized, or delayed. Your recognition of pain underlies the Stop, Caution, Go system to treating injuries.

What Causes Injuries?

The first step in managing injuries is preventing them in the first place, or at least lessening their severity. Knowing how to reduce your chances of suffering an injury is a key to maintaining good health and to understanding sports medicine. Understanding and remembering these four factors that contribute to sports injuries can be very helpful:

- Change
- Alignment
- Twisting
- Speed

The more factors that are combined, the higher the risk for injury.

Change

The human body does not like sudden change. Overuse injuries occur when there is a sudden increase or change in training technique. Most injuries occur in spring, when there is a dramatic increase in the amount and frequency of sport participation. Here is a good rule of thumb: Do not increase the distance, frequency, or duration of your training program by more than 10 percent a week. The human body has wonderful adaptive power and potential—if given enough time to adapt.

Alignment

Alignment means "arrangement in a straight line." Well-aligned athletes—those born with straight legs, straight spines, and straight arms—have fewer injuries. People who have slight spine curvatures, bowed legs, or knock knees are more susceptible to injury. Young women who have wide hips and knock knees injure their kneecaps more frequently than others. Middle-aged men who become more bowlegged commonly develop knee problems. Throwing athletes, who produce more outward angulation of the arm at the elbow, are prone to elbow and shoulder injuries.

Sometimes there is little you can do if you are not born with straight alignment. In rare cases extensive bone surgery can be performed. A podiatrist can put inserts in your shoes, which may help manage the alignment problem. The important thing to remember if you know you have poor alignment is to be very careful with the intensity of your approach to sports. You should consult your physician about your specific concerns.

Twisting

The human body evolved primarily as a straight locomotion system for running, not for high-intensity twisting maneuvers like those performed in volleyball, basketball, or gymnastics. Though twisting may help you reach your athletic goal, it also increases the likelihood that you will be injured.

Speed

When it comes to speed, the human body can be compared to a car. The more often you drive your car and the faster you drive it, the more likely it is that you will have an accident and that the accident will be serious. The faster you run, bicycle, or swim, and the more you do these activities, the more you will stress the musculoskeletal system and the more opportunity you have for injury.

The worst scenario is a springtime athlete who, after being inactive all winter, suddenly starts exercising and has three or four factors combining to create problems. The athlete may suddenly increase the amount of exercise (change), have bowed legs (alignment), twist suddenly, and then increase speed. This athlete is very susceptible to injuries. If you are aware of these four factors, you will undoubtedly prevent most injuries from happening to you.

Types of Injuries

There are basically two types of injuries: acute and chronic. Using a burn as an example, you can injure yourself very badly either by putting your hand directly into a fire—resulting in an acute injury—or by overexposing yourself to the sun and burning—a chronic overuse injury. Both types of injuries can be severe and can be classified by degrees: first degree, second degree, or third degree—third degree being the worst type of injury. These kinds of injuries are explained in more detail in the following sections.

Acute Traumatic Injuries

When you watch professional football and see someone's knee being severely twisted and dislocated, that is an obvious acute injury. In an acute injury, muscles and ligaments are severely torn and bones may be fractured. These injuries produce a great deal of pain and swelling and require immediate first aid and referral to an emergency room.

Chronic Overuse Injuries

Most people clearly understand the treatment of an acute injury, namely, go see the doctor, rest, and avoid exercising the injured area. However, chronic overuse injuries can be just as severe but are often ignored. Stress fracture or arthritis can be developing. Athletes sometimes try to "run out the pain," and the result is more injury. The principle of listening to your body is very important with overuse injuries. Chronic overuse injuries are best treated by reducing activity, choosing alternative activities, treating the inflammation if appropriate, exercising properly, and using common sense.

Reducing activity is important because the main cause of an overuse injury is usually a sudden change and then a sudden acceleration in activity. As with a burn, reducing inflammation is one of the key treatments. You should consider applying ice, immobilizing the injured area, and using anti-inflammatory medications such as aspirin or ibuprofen. Just as we may sit in the sun ignoring the sunburn that is developing, we sometimes don't realize the extent of an injury and continue to expose ourselves. When a biker or runner who has a sore knee keeps pushing because the pain is minimal, problems can develop. Again, the most important principle here is to listen to your body and go with caution. There is no need to stop activity completely. Choosing alternative activities and reducing activity is common sense.

Most overuse injuries occur with twisting activities common in ball sports. During periods of pain, apply the Stop, Caution, Go concept (explained in more detail in the next section) by reducing the twisting activities and progressively increasing activities that keep you moving forward, activities such as biking, running, and swimming. As pain subsides, you can gradually return to twisting sports. Work on muscle development, addressing the factors of flexibility, endurance, strength, and speed. These factors will be explained further under the Rehab Exercises (see pp. 23-25).

This has been a brief summary of types of injuries and general approaches in treating them. The 40 Specific Injury Treatments in Part III of this book will help you establish, for specific injuries, a plan using these overall concepts. The next section explains the Stop, Caution, Go concept on which this book is based.

Stop, Caution, Go: Learning to Listen to Your Body

In our clinic, all exercise is assigned one of three colors symbolizing activity levels and other approaches to treatment. Each of the 40 Specific Injury Treatments in

Part III has a stop and go light, which indicates the appropriate activity level. When considering activity levels, these colors are guidelines.

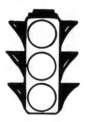

RED means avoid hard use. Reduce activity.

YELLOW means be cautious. Let pain be your guide.

GREEN means full use is fine. Listen to your body.

For instance, if your particular injury is labeled Red, you should slow down from your normal activity level, either stopping or reducing activity almost completely. If your injury is labeled Yellow, you should be cautious about approaching activity and let pain guide your level of activity. When it hurts, slow down or stop. If your activity is labeled Green, then you can pursue activity at your normal pace—full speed ahead—though you should always listen to your body for any signs of problems.

The key concept is that you should go with caution and moderation and avoid excessive pain while exercising. Identify your own strengths and weaknesses as they apply to your particular sport. For instance, if you are a gymnast you are probably already sufficiently flexible, but you may need work on strength. If you are a marathon runner, you probably already have great endurance, but your performance may be enhanced by work on speed, flexibility, and strength. If you are a weightlifter, you are already strong but may need to spend more time on endurance and flexibility. With commitment and a plan, you can balance these factors in yourself and find your activities more successful and less likely to result in injuries. Later, Part III looks at exercise alternatives for specific injuries or conditions.

The 6-Point Condition Summary

Before considering a treatment plan, it is essential that you have a proper diagnosis from a health care professional. You should have enough information so that you can work with the professional to establish a specific treatment plan. The 40 Specific Injury Treatments in Part III of this book include a 6-Point Condition Summary. The following six points are covered for each condition:

1. Definition
2. Cause
3. Subjective symptoms
4. Objective findings

5. Testing procedures
6. Prognosis

These six points combine to give you a description of the condition, and this description is complete enough to develop a specific treatment plan.

1. Definition

A brief description of the key characteristics of the injury, including its location, anatomy, symptoms, and cause.

2. Cause

Medical conditions are classified by various types of causes. Types of causes are listed here. The first three are the most common causes of sports injuries; however, the other causes, though rare, should be kept in mind:

Traumatic—the most frequent cause of sports injuries.

Degenerative—the middle-aged athlete is susceptible to "wear and tear" as the cause of pain.

Mechanical—a loose fragment in a joint could be causing pain. A pinched nerve can be from a mechanical cause.

Vascular—blood vessel block or obstruction should always be ruled out as a cause of pain in an extremity.

Tumor—a rare cause of pain in an athlete, but a tumor is one reason an X-ray should be taken in all painful conditions.

Infection—the pain and swelling of a joint could be from infection rather than inflammation.

Psychogenic—sometimes the stress and frustration of sports causes mental discomfort.

Congenital—this is a rare but possible cause of pain in an extremity and comes from a birth defect of a bone or joint.

Metabolic—poor performance in an athlete could be from an endocrine or fluid imbalance rather than an injury.

Allergic—poor performance in sports could be from an allergy such as asthma.

3. Subjective Symptoms

What you as a patient perceive and should describe to your health care provider. See "Working With Your Physician" in Part I for further description.

4. Objective Findings

What the physician perceives and detects through examination. See "Working With Your Physician" in Part I for further description.

5. Testing Procedures

These are the specialized tests that can range from simple X-rays to sophisticated surgical procedures such as arthroscopy. A list and explanations of possible tests follow:

X-rays (Roentgenograms)—These "photos" are produced by an X-ray machine that takes a picture generally of a bony structure of your body. X-rays are extremely helpful in diagnosing bone injuries and fractures. They have limited value in showing soft tissue injuries in muscle, ligament, or cartilage. X-rays should be taken in almost all sports injuries to rule out other congenital and tumor conditions that sometimes are being masked by the sports injury.

Bone Scan (Radionuclide)—This test is used for the detection and localization of bone lesions and inflammation around a joint such as arthritis. A radioactive material is injected into the blood stream. Two or three hours later, the patient is "scanned" under a computerized sensor to measure the uptake of the material at the bone and joint level. A bone scan is a very sensitive test and is used to indicate bone turnover and reaction. A patient with a possible fracture may have a completely normal X-ray but a very "hot" bone scan.

Thermogram—This is a heat photograph using special crystal and infrared scanning equipment to measure human body surface temperature. It creates a color picture in an attempt to provide objective evidence of the pain. In our practice, we do not use thermograms; however, they are available at some facilities using high-intensity computer equipment. We find thermograms of limited value.

Arthrogram—This is an X-ray study in which a radiopaque dye (which appears dense on an X-ray) is injected into the joint—generally the knee or the shoulder. If there is a tear in the tendon (shoulder) or the meniscus (knee), the arthrogram can be very helpful in detecting this lesion. The technique is technically demanding, and the results may vary with the experience of the radiologist. At our hospital, we have an extremely reliable arthrogram system, and we find them to be 90 to 95 percent accurate.

Myelogram—This form of the X-ray is taken of the spine after injecting a radiopaque material into the dural sac of the spine. This is an excellent test for showing a herniated lumbar disc but generally is not performed unless the pain is severe and surgery is being contemplated.

MRI (Magnetic Resonance Imaging)—This test, developed during the 1980s, produces a "photo" in response to the protons and their electromagnetic force in each tissue. The result produces a significant contrast between abnormal tissue and healthy tissue. The test is becoming more available but is very expensive. Prior insurance company approval is generally recommended. In sports injuries, the test is helpful in finding tears of the knee ligament such as the anterior cruciate ligament, a torn rotator cuff, or a torn meniscus of the knee.

CAT Scan (Computerized Axial Tomography)—The word "tomogram" comes from the Latin root *tomus*, which means "to cut." Using special computerized techniques, various nonsurgical "cuts" taken with the X-ray beam can produce localized pictures of the anatomy. The various X-ray cuts are integrated with a computer and produce a picture that is extremely accurate for spine lesions and various bone and joint problems.

EMG (Electromyogram)—This is an electrical study of the muscle to determine various muscle diseases due to nerve and spinal injuries. Several weeks after an injury to a nerve, diagnostic electrical impulses can be recorded in the muscle. These impulses are very helpful in making the proper diagnosis of a muscle and nerve injury.

EKG (Electrocardiogram)—Though not specifically a sports medicine test for musculoskeletal injuries, the EKG done as a cardiac stress test can be very helpful for an athlete's rehabilitation and for determining cardiovascular fitness.

Arthroscopy—This surgical technique, developed during the 1970s, was initially a diagnostic test to evaluate the internal structures of a joint. The test now is refined and, with small scopes, can be used for the elbow and wrist. Most often this is done with general anesthesia. Small incisions are made and a telescope about the diameter of a pencil is inserted into the joint to give direct visualization of cartilage, ligaments, and meniscus lesions. This test is very accurate but should not be used until more traditional diagnostic techniques, such as a history and physical, routine X-rays, and perhaps an arthrogram or an MRI, have been performed. The advantage of the arthroscope is that after the diagnostic procedure is performed, certain surgical procedures such as removing cartilage lesions or repairing injured ligaments can also be performed through the arthroscope.

These tests can be expensive and very confusing. However, they are helpful in integrating the history and physical in order to arrive at a specific diagnosis and treatment plan for an injured athlete. Your health care provider helps to correlate and integrate your history, your physical condition, and your diagnosis and then determines which test you need. Once these steps are completed, you are ready for a treatment plan. (The next section explains the 10 steps in a typical 10-Point Treatment Plan.)

6. Prognosis

This is the final step in describing a condition and provides a general guideline about what will happen as a result of this injury. You need to realize that medicine is not an exact science, and each case tends to act differently, though there are obvious similarities within injury categories. A health care provider does not have a crystal ball. The word *prognosis* comes from the Latin words *pro*, meaning "before," and *gnoscere*, meaning "to come to know." Based on the physician's experience and years of management and knowledge, the health professional may be able to "know before" the end result actually occurs. But remember, medicine is not an exact science.

The 10-Point Treatment Plan

The 10-Point Treatment Plan looks at 10 key aspects of treating an injury:

1. Activity levels
2. Alternative activities
3. Rehab exercises
4. Support
5. Thermal treatment
6. Medication
7. Equipment
8. Nutrition
9. Fluids
10. Surfaces

When you are listening and then responding to your body, these 10 items are all very important. This section will focus on each of them in detail. In Part III, specific sports injuries and conditions are explained by looking at a 6-Point Condition Summary and then a 10-Point Treatment Plan that can be applied to each condition.

1. Activity Levels

Of the 10 areas covered in the 10-Point Treatment Plan, activity is the most important because it relates directly to the Stop, Caution, and Go concept. In the

40 Specific Injury Treatments, activity levels are designated by a stoplight with red meaning Stop; yellow meaning Caution; or green meaning Go.

Coaches, especially in football, are familiar with the concept of "red shirting." This is for the injured athlete who may participate but should avoid any strenuous contact or hitting maneuvers. Our clinic uses the concept of "yellow shirting," which means Go With Caution or let pain be your guide, again supporting the concept of listening to your body.

As previously discussed, you will have to learn the what, how, and who of listening for pain. There are different kinds of pain, and each warrants a different response or a different level of activity. The real dilemma in sports and fitness is knowing how to differentiate among these types of pain. Activity Levels in the 10-Point Treatment Plan guide you toward the right activity level based on the kind of pain you have.

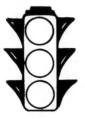

RED Avoid hard use

YELLOW "Let pain be the guide"

GREEN "Listen to your body"

Types of Pain

One type of pain is that vague pain you may experience in your large muscle groups during and after muscle exercise. This pain is probably due to a buildup of lactic acid and is a typical characteristic of a training effect. Vague pain suggests that you should simply reduce activities but not necessarily change your training program. The basic approach with vague pain is to listen to your body. In this case, yellow or Caution may be the activity level most appropriate. If you feel that you are improving and feeling better with increasing activity, then continue with that more moderate approach.

Realize that you can be fooled and that the vague ache in your thigh may not be muscle but rather nerve pain from a herniated disc, which can be greatly aggravated by activity. If there is any question, reduce rather than increase activities. Again, here is where a diagnosis by a health professional is very important to help you differentiate between nerve pain, vascular pain, and muscle pain. When exercising with nerve pain, it is important to concentrate on straight activities (see "Alternative Activities," pp. 21-23) and avoid hard, sudden twisting activities.

A second type of pain is localized. It indicates a more serious problem and is located directly on the tendon, bone, joint, or ligament. You can usually put your finger right on it and say, "It hurts here." Localized pain suggests a more serious injury around the joint and probably means that your training program has gone too fast or too hard. The main treatment in this situation is a significant reduction in your activities. The familiar saying "No pain, no gain" is simply not correct for localized pain.

One of the advantages of being an experienced athlete is that you've gone through the risks and injuries of sports and know that sometimes injuries don't completely heal, or they take a long time to heal and lead to permanent changes in your body. The young, immature athlete doesn't have these experiences until injuries have already occurred. Some of the risks of abusing and using an inflamed, painful joint include permanent damage such as arthritis, torn meniscus, torn tendons, and stress fractures.

Delayed pain is a third kind of pain you may encounter. When planning your activity level, you should be aware of the possibility of delayed pain such as that caused by overuse to a joint that doesn't hurt for 24 hours. Arthritis pain or *chondromalacia* of the knee doesn't give you immediate feedback. You can be injuring yourself but not feel it until a day or so later, and this can be frustrating. Here, careful monitoring is vital. Keep reducing activity until pain is at a minimal level. Don't exercise hard 2 days in a row—follow a hard day with a light day in order to give yourself time to rest and recover.

2. Alternative Activities

Choosing alternative activities is an important aspect of treating most injuries. Consequently, alternative activities are an important point in any effective treatment plan. Though sometimes the best treatment for a painful joint or muscle is to Stop all activities and rest completely, there are a number of major complications that can occur from the abrupt halt of all activities—cardiovascular deconditioning, muscle atrophy, increased body fat, mental depression, and occasionally bone loss or osteoporosis. The secret is to treat the entire body, not just the painful area. The best treatment plan is moderation and listening to your body.

At our clinic, we classify activities into three zones:

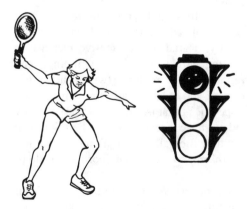

RED Hard twisting activities— basketball, volleyball, racquetball, wrestling, football, soccer

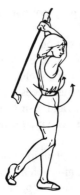

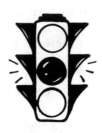

YELLOW Moderate twisting activities—dancing, tennis, bowling, golf, skiing

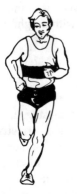

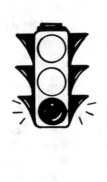

GREEN Straight activities—race walking, swimming, biking, jogging, running, running in a swimming pool, cross-country skiing, jumping rope

You should keep in mind that another factor in these classifications is intensity. Some activities have the potential for being either high or low impact. For instance, an activity such as aerobic dancing, though usually classified at the yellow or cautious level of activity, can actually be at any of the three levels depending on the intensity of participation.

From our years of experience in treating fitness and sports injuries, we have found that the athlete/patient will not accept the advice to stop all activities and rest. During the rehabilitation of an injury, a gradual, progressive increase in activity level should be permitted, starting with walking or swimming, then progressing to biking or running and eventually to the moderate twisting activities, and progressing eventually to hard twisting activities, usually the ball sports.

Generally, sports injuries are "sport specific"; that is, injuries occur primarily in one sport. The basketball player tends to have a recurrence of the injuries in basketball but will be able to play softball or football with minimal difficulties. Very simply, if you are having pain with one sport, switch sports. You don't necessarily have to stop all sports.

There are many considerations when choosing an alternative activity. Your choice may be based in part on how competitive you are in the sport you normally pursue. Do you want to risk the deconditioning of the muscles you usually use for the sake of ongoing activity? The choice is up to you. Just be sure you consider your goals and try to stay active if that is the recommendation of your treatment plan.

3. Rehab Exercises

Rehabilitation exercises are the specific exercises you pursue to condition your injured muscles so that you can return to your regular sport as a full participant. Rehab exercises are an integral part of a treatment plan and are in addition to any other activity or alternative activity as explained earlier. Muscles have four important qualities (also known as FESS), which can be enhanced with exercise:

- Flexibility
- Endurance
- Strength
- Speed

Even the best athletes who naturally have these qualities developed at a high level usually have room for improvement in one area or another.

Some athletes have great flexibility but lack endurance or strength. A marathon runner may have fantastic endurance but may lack strength and flexibility. Heavy weightlifters may have tremendous strength but may lack flexibility and endurance. The list of strengths and weaknesses can go on and on for each sport (see Table 2.1).

The question often arises: Which is more important, flexibility, endurance, speed, or strength? The answer is this: Only you know. Listen to your body. Ask yourself: Are you stiff? Are you weak? Are you winded? Are you slow? The goal for fitness enthusiasts and athletes is to identify their strengths and

Table 2.1 Qualities of Muscle for Selected Sports

Sport	Flexibility	Endurance	Strength	Speed
Gymnastics	+	o	o	o
Marathon running	o	+	o	o
Weight lifting	o	o	+	o
100-yard dash	o	o	o	+
Basketball (professional)	+	+	+	+

+ indicates more important quality

o indicates less important quality

weaknesses, particularly as they relate to activities the athletes would like to pursue. When areas needing improvement are identified, an exercise plan can be established. For the athlete needing work in all areas, we suggest the following order of importance: strength, endurance, flexibility, speed.

The guidelines for rehab exercises follow:

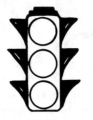

RED Avoid a hard, bouncing stretch; avoid vigorously bent joint with weights
YELLOW Moderate stretch; moderately bent joint with weights
GREEN Light stretch; joint straight with weights

Flexibility training can be helpful but may be the area that is overemphasized the most. It is even possible to become too flexible if you go beyond range of motion for a particular joint, and this opens up the possibility of more injuries. If there is any question, spend more of your time on strength than flexibility.

Stretching

An important part of an exercise or activity program is stretching. Listen to your body for indications of when to stretch. If you are feeling tight, then that is an indication that you should stretch. If you feel tight primarily before you exercise, then that is the time to stretch. On the other hand, if you feel tight after you exercise, then that is the time to stretch. There are, however, specific guidelines that relate to stretching, and they are important to follow.

In our office, we tend to see more people who hurt themselves while stretching than people who hurt themselves while doing strengthening exercises. You should always make sure your muscles are warmed up before starting stretching exercises. Note that warming up doesn't mean stretching. It means making sure your muscles are warm before beginning stretching. This means inducing a light sweat either by external heat (steam, hot pad, etc.) or by light activity (run, pitch, etc.). Once your muscles are warm, start with static stretches, which do not go beyond the range of your joints. You should hold these stretches 6 to 8 seconds and repeat them 3 to 10 times per day.

Athletes are most likely to be hurt when there is an imbalance between flexibility, endurance, strength, and speed. Olympic gold medal winners, professional athletes, and world champions are blessed with high development in all these areas, but they have also learned how to balance their abilities. Your goal as an athlete or fitness enthusiast is to identify your areas of weakness and concentrate on improving those areas through proper muscle development, endurance, and aerobic training.

It takes motivation to establish a regular exercise program aimed at rehabilitating muscles and developing these four qualities. The ideal is to be self-motivated enough to train and exercise without the need of special equipment, trainers, coaches, or physical therapists; however, the reality is that most athletes do need help—from a physician, trainer, coach, or physical therapist. You should look for help in identifying areas for improvement and for help in providing appropriate incentives and in setting goals. Sometimes it is easier to be motivated when you are in a class or group with others who have similar goals. It is a rare person who can remain motivated all alone in a cold, damp basement while lifting weights or timing the minutes on an exercise bike. The key, as we have said throughout this book, is to listen to your body. When your body tells you it needs exercise, that should be enough motivation for most committed athletes.

Exercises Using Equipment

Three standard types of conditioning exercises involve equipment. Isometrics refers to keeping the joint straight and adding variable resistance. An example of this kind of exercise is straight-leg-raising exercises with weights on the shin. These exercises are good for situations in which full range of motion is painful. Isotonics are the standard weight-lifting procedures that combine progressive resistant exercises with joint motion. Equipment includes barbells and weight machines such as Nautilus and Universal. Isokinetic machines have fixed speed and a variable resistance with an accommodating resistance. An example of this is the Cybex. The isokinetic machines are excellent for rehabilitation of injured knee ligaments, such as the anterior cruciate, if no pain is produced.

The Stop, Caution, Go concept is also applied to rehabilitation exercises. Red means the hard stretching and vigorous bent-joint activities with weights; you should avoid these if you are injured. Yellow means moderate stretching and bent-joint activities with light weights; you can do these activities with caution after you listen to your body. Green means light stretching and straight-joint exercises with light weights. These are the exercises that should be performed early in the rehabilitation process when the joint is still sore. For example, if the ankle and knee are painful, do your exercises without moving the joint (isometric). Putting simple elastic tubing and light weights on the shin and foot will allow you to exercise joints such as the hip without experiencing pain at the ankle.

The illustrations in Part IV demonstrate how many of these exercises can be performed. These exercises have been used successfully by thousands of athletes at our sports medicine clinic. In the final analysis, go with caution and moderation. Avoid exercises that cause excessive pain. Identify your own strengths and weaknesses as they apply to your particular sport.

4. Support

Braces, bandages, and tape around inflamed muscles and joints can be used for temporary support and stabilization. The ''best'' support is your normal muscle development. If you want to build support and think you need a brace, start by developing strong muscles. Until you have proper muscle and joint stability, however, it is certainly advisable to purchase and wear a brace.

Types of Braces

For the knee, which is the most commonly braced joint, your choices for a brace are from the following list:

- Simple elastic bandage ($5)
- Elastic pull-on ($10)
- Neoprene elastic pull-on ($40)
- Knit, with metal hinges ($60)
- Complex patella stabilizing ($60)
- Semi-custom-made plastic and metal stabilizing ($300 off the shelf)
- Custom-made, metal and plastic hinge ($500–$700)

The selection of a knee brace can be a very complex task and is frequently confusing for both the patient and the health care provider. Here again, listen to your body to give you guidance. If you are doing hard pivoting, twisting, and jumping sports and feel that your knee is going out of place, your physician may prescribe a high-tech brace for the diagnosis of a torn ligament. There is no guarantee that these braces will correct the problem, but they can be very helpful when combined with cautious exercise and adequate muscle rehabilitation. The brace may not cure you, and you may need surgery. For moderate, simple activities, less expensive braces can certainly do the job. Many of these braces may be partly reimbursed by your insurance if they are prescribed by a physician.

Braces for Everyone?

There is a great deal of controversy about the "prophylactic" use of braces, especially in high school football. Not only has it not been proven that braces help prevent football injuries, but the cost can be overwhelming. Assuming you have 40 players, each of whom is using a $500 brace, the cost to the school is $20,000. That same $20,000 could be used to hire a trainer who would help the team much more than a closet full of braces.

As in all aspects of medicine, particular braces should be used for selected problems in certain instances. A brace should not be used as an excuse not to exercise your muscles.

One of the major advantages of a brace is that it becomes a visual symbol to the other players and coaches—a symbol that you have a problem. Nobody likes to admit to having a sore knee or to ask for help or less stress; however, simply by putting a brace on your knee or your elbow, you are saying, "Take it easy, I need help. I am listening to my body." However, don't look for a "quick fix" with a brace. Braces are not a panacea for all joint problems. Braces, as with medications, have benefits, risks, and complications. Support guidelines follow:

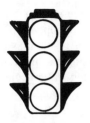

RED Cast

YELLOW Elastic sleeve, brace

GREEN Simple elastic wrap

5. Thermal Treatment

This term refers to the application of heat or cold to an injury. Though many first aid manuals suggest using ice for the first 24 to 48 hours after an injury and then recommend switching to heat, injured people seem to mistakenly remember the word *heat* more often than the word *ice*. The general rule is that localized pain or any localized swelling should be treated with ice. The red, yellow, and green classifications for thermal treatment are as follows:

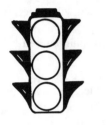

RED Avoid hot packs

YELLOW Lukewarm soaks

GREEN Ice packs

Short of a severely dislocated joint or fractured bone, which require emergency treatment, the initial treatment of acute traumatic injuries is reflected in the acronym RICE, a familiar term to most athletes. RICE means

R   Rest
I   Ice
C   Compression
E   Elevation

A burn is again very helpful in illustrating the treatment of a sports injury. With an acute burn of the hand, there is an initial injury of tissue, outpouring of fluids, and damage to the capillaries, all resulting in swelling—the inflammatory process. The initial treatment is by RICE to reduce swelling and to rest tissues. Think of a sports injury as a burn. Immediately take the injured area ''out-of-the-fire,'' and apply ice. More detail on ice is presented in the next section. Rest reduces tissue damage and persistent inflammation by immobilizing the injured area. Rest can range from reduced activity to a complete immobilization of the injured area by, for instance, a leg cast. Compression means wrapping the injured area so that tissue pressure is maintained and the injured area and injured joint or muscle are immobilized. You should be careful not to apply too much compression because constriction of the blood vessels can result in vascular complications. Elevation means reducing swelling by raising the injured area above the heart or simply lying down and keeping the leg or arm elevated. Elevation is appropriate during initial periods of pain and swelling.

Ice Is Nice

Ice is the key component of RICE. Ice is an extremely effective initial treatment for most sports injuries: It acts as a local anesthetic to help relieve pain and also helps enhance the flow of blood from the skin to the deeper tissues for healing. It is a mistake, in fact, to treat an injury initially with heat because it causes more swelling and inflammation. Some trainers use the concept PIE, which stands for Pressure, Ice, and Elevation. In this school of thought, the previous words *rest* and *compression* are replaced with the concept of pressure. Thus, the trainer will use an iced bandage that is immediately wrapped around an injured area. The result will be a reduced outpouring of fluid—less edema.

Another effective way to use ice is in a styrofoam cup filled with water, frozen, and left in a freezer. The ice in the cup (you may need to peel away some of the cup to expose the ice) can be used as a local massage for pain caused by local tendinitis, tennis elbow, or ankle sprain.

Ice should be considered a medication that has a prescribed dose and frequency of use. Generally, 10 or 15 minutes of an ice bath or local ice pack is all the skin can tolerate. Ice can be used three or four times a day, but, as is the case with any medication, complications may develop if it's overused.

I am reminded of the case of a basketball player who injured his ankle in a game. The coach directed him to keep his ankle in an ice bucket for 2 full days nonstop. After a while, the ice became an anesthetic and the pain disappeared; however, the ice continued to have an effect. After 40 hours, the circulation in the player's foot stopped. Gangrene developed and the player's forefoot and toes had to be amputated—a tragic and definitely avoidable event. Like anything in life and medicine, too much of a good thing can be more dangerous than the original problem.

Switching From Ice to Heat

Knowing when to switch from ice to heat is based on the principle of how to listen to your body. As the local pain, tenderness, and swelling gradually subside and the symptoms change to tightness and stiffness, you can start to loosen the muscle with warm soaks and local heat application.

Heat is good for loosening the muscles in the large muscle groups around the thigh, back, and shoulders. The general rule is to use heat before activity and ice after the activity. If you are ever in the locker room of a professional baseball team, observe the pitchers. Hot packs are applied around the shoulder and elbow for an hour or two before the game. The arm is kept warm in a thick jacket. The pitcher then performs, keeping the pitching arm warm with a jacket during the game. Immediately after the game, the trainer will put the elbow into an ice whirlpool or ice bucket to reduce pain, inflammation, and swelling.

Many people, even athletes, do not understand this principle of applying heat before and ice or cold after an activity. For instance, at most health clubs you will see people sitting in the sauna, steam room, or hot whirlpool after the racquetball or tennis game. The process should probably be reversed. You should warm up in the sauna for about 5 minutes before your activity. Afterward, you don't need to warm up, but that's when most people do it. Of course, you can warm up too much and find yourself exhausted before you even start to exercise. That's why 5 minutes of warm-up is usually sufficient.

For general discomfort and tightness, heat is most effective for the large muscle groups around the thigh, trunk, shoulders, back, and neck. There are no absolute rules for the application of heat, and it can be used in combination or contrast with ice. Try 10 minutes of heat, followed by 5 minutes of ice massage, followed by another 10 minutes of heat. The contrast may alter blood flow and enhance healing.

When deciding whether to apply heat or ice, be flexible, consider various approaches, and listen to your body. If ice is not working, then switch to heat. If heat is not working, then switch to ice. Combining the two may be very effective. Always keep in mind that overdoing heat or ice may result in complications that can be worse than the original injury.

6. Medication

Medications are potentially part of most treatment plans, and they lend themselves nicely to the red, yellow, and green classifications.

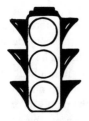

RED Avoid high doses and excessive quantities of medications, vitamins, or minerals.
YELLOW You may take prescribed anti-inflammatory medications, such as ibuprofen and possible local steroid injections.
GREEN You may take over-the-counter medications such as aspirin or Tylenol—two with meals.

Different Approaches to Medications

Medications are helpful for two reasons—to relieve pain and to reduce local inflammation. There are two extreme attitudes toward medications. One group of people consists of individuals who are purists or naturalists and avoid any form of medication. The other group consists of people who are looking for a "quick fix" and take excessive quantities of minerals, vitamins, and anti-inflammatory medication in hopes of curing the condition. The cautious approach is one of moderation and listening to your body, which might include taking minimal doses of anti-inflammatory medication.

As with most aspects of a treatment plan, there are problems with either extreme. You may experience complications by not taking medication when it is warranted; however, you will also experience complications by taking excessive medications. Sometimes a little help in the form of pain relief and anti-inflammatory relief is needed during the rehabilitation process, but somewhere you need to find a happy medium. This can usually be accomplished by letting your body indicate what levels of medication produce the best results and can be tolerated. There are no fixed rules when it comes to medication.

Anti-Inflammatory and Over-the-Counter Medications

Nonsteroidal, anti-inflammatory drugs act by changing the local chemistry at the inflamed site through various modes of action. A full discussion of medications is beyond the scope of this book; however, you should be aware of some of the over-the-counter, nonprescription drugs such as aspirin or ibuprofen. At 200 mg, ibuprofen (brand names Advil, Motrin, etc.) does not need a prescription. However, at 400, 600, and 800 mg, ibuprofen, including Indocin, Motrin, Nalfon, Naprosyn, Rufen, and Voltaren, to name a few, requires a prescription from a doctor. Most of the strong anti-inflammatory medications can have a major side effect—stomach and gastrointestinal upset. We tell patients that 1 in 100 patients on these medications may develop a gastric ulcer. One way to reduce local stomach irritation is by taking a new prescription product called Carafate, a stomach protector, but you should discuss this with your physician first. You must balance the rewards of taking any medication with the potential complications and risks. Again, the principle is to listen to your body.

Anti-Inflammatory Injection

The product we use in our office is called Kenalog. It is a crystal steroid product related to cortisone. Cortisone is a naturally occurring substance made in the body to help fight stress and inflammation and to promote healing. The medication helps to relieve local inflammation such as tendinitis, synovitis, and localized arthritis. Occasionally, the injection is used as a "test" for inflammation versus mechanical tear. If the pain rapidly subsides and is relieved, the pain was probably from an inflammation. If pain persists, the pain may be from a mechanical tear.

The mechanism of action or how the injection works is to reduce inflammation, promote healing, and decrease scar formation. A possible side effect, in a dark-skinned person, may be local depigmentation and whitening of the skin. There may be a temporary weakening of the injected tendon. Therefore, caution in hard jumping is recommended for about 2 to 4 weeks after the injection. Frequent injections, more than two or three a year, are not recommended.

Local pain and swelling sometimes follow the injection. If there is a local flareup, you should limit activity, and you may apply ice and take aspirin for 1 or 2 days. Anti-inflammatory injections should not be abused and should not be a substitute for common sense and modification of activity. As with all medications, there are risks and rewards, and you should discuss them with your physician. In our practice, we have found that one local injection of steroid in and around an inflamed joint that has not responded to treatment is a safe approach compared to the potential complications of more aggressive treatment such as surgery.

7. Equipment

As part of rehabilitation or training, exercise equipment is very important for cardiovascular and musculoskeletal development. The list of possible equipment you can buy includes treadmill, trampoline, cross-country ski machine, bicycle, stair-climbing apparatus, rowing machine, and weight-lifting equipment (free weights and isotonic machines). Other equipment is available for purchase; however, these are the most common and most useful pieces of equipment available.

Patients and athletes are frequently overwhelmed by the multitude of equipment. Your decision depends on many factors—availability, cost, space, and personal objectives and motivation. Here again, the principle of listening to your body should dictate which equipment to buy; however, there are other alternatives to buying expensive equipment. One is to join a health club, where all of this equipment is there for you to use. You can also perform many effective exercises yourself with such simple materials as sandbags and rubber tubing. The treatment plan that has evolved for many patients in our clinic includes the use of free weights—sandbags of 3, 5, and 10 pounds that can be applied to the arm or leg for strength training. Rubber tubing can then be used for flexibility training and strengthening.

The red, yellow, and green classifications for equipment are as follows:

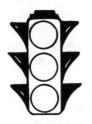 **RED** Avoid vigorous stair climbing
Avoid strenuous weight lifting
YELLOW Rowing, trampoline
Moderate weight lifting
GREEN Treadmill, bike, cross-country skiing

Equipment Choices

The following explanations are based on the assumption that you are planning to buy equipment for your home and that you need to make the right choices.

Treadmills. Through the 1980s, the cost of electric treadmills has gradually come down to where they can be afforded by the average consumer willing to spend between $500 and $1,000. Some very sophisticated treadmills can cost between $3,000 and $5,000, but these are generally not necessary for the average athlete. Certain considerations are weight, noise, and ability to change incline and speed. At about the $1,000 range, an electric treadmill can give you many of the features and the durability that you need.

Even though running on a treadmill seems to simulate normal running and walking, it is not the case. The floor is moving rapidly against your foot. This can sometimes aggravate minor pain around the front of the knee in the region of the patella. The aggravation is generally brief but is a reason to go slowly and moderately. During your first few days with the equipment you might tend to push yourself as hard as possible and ignore minor problems. This can lead to endless frustration from pain, and eventually you stop using your $1,000 toy.

Trampoline. For the person who wants to run in place and maximize shock absorption, a spring-suspended trampoline can be an excellent choice. The aerobic benefit is minimal, but there is very little shock. This offers an excellent alternative at a low cost. Lack of motivation and boredom become factors to consider.

Cross-Country Ski Machine. An indoor cross-country ski machine has been available for many years. Several inexpensive copies of the original have become available. Just as cross-country skiing provides excellent upper- and lower-body exercise, so do cross-country machines. Sometimes the twisting of the upper body can produce low back and neck discomfort.

Bicycle. Stationary bicycles have been available for many years. One of the concerns is that they are too upright and do not have the same handlebar-to-seat alignment ratios as a regular outdoor touring bicycle. An approach to this problem is to take a mountain bike and purchase a wind trainer, which is a stand to put on the rear wheel for basement and home use. This gives you the best of both worlds. You have a year-round bicycle for outdoor biking and indoor biking at a moderate price. This way you are assured of having an indoor bicycle that fits your body frame.

Many of the bicycles at clubs, even though they are adjustable, are rarely adjusted for your body size. This is a frequent cause of neck, back, and knee complaints in the club bicyclist. Other indoor bicycle alternatives feature a large oscillating fan on the front wheel. This large front wheel is also controlled by reciprocally moving handlebars. This gives you the ability to exercise both your arms and your legs at the same time. An advantage is that you can still exercise your upper body yet also rest and protect a painful knee or ankle if necessary.

Stair-Climbing Apparatus. In recent years stair-climbing machines have become progressively popular. These machines can give rapid aerobic exercise in a short amount of time. In our clinic, we are finding increasing numbers of patients with knee complaints, especially about the patella, because of stair-climbing machines. Since stair climbing in general causes many knee problems, so will the stair-climbing machine. If you start slowly and moderately and progress at a gradual rate, it can be very safe exercise. However, people on the machines tend to put a great deal of force on their upper arms and sway their backs in a very unnatural fashion, which can lead to low back pain. Since there is no air motion (fan), overheating and dehydration can be a problem.

Rowing Machines. Rowing machines have been very popular for the last 20 years. One of the most popular features a large flywheel, which produces wind resistance and excellent cooling for the rower. Excessive knee bending and back flexion can occur with rowing; rowing should, therefore, be used in moderation for patients with knee and back problems.

Weight-Lifting Equipment. The weight lifter has two choices—either free weights or isotonic weight machines. In our clinic, we start patients with simple 5- to 10-pound sandbags that can be wrapped around the calf, thigh, or arm to gradually build up flexibility, endurance, speed, and strength (see previous Section 3, "Rehab Exercises"). From free weights, you can progress to dumb-bells, which may have some advantages over machines. Dumbbell weights train your ability to coordinate your muscles with added balance and resistance, while the isotonic machines (Universal, Nautilus) offer excellent resistance through the full range of motion but do not train your coordination and balance. The machine weights can especially aggravate patellar problems because of the added resistance when the knee is flexed. The rule here is to go gradually and moderately and avoid excessive flexion. Listen to your body. If pain is developing around the joint, change the routine to other joints. "Circuit training" is an excellent aerobic exercise in which you move from station to station perhaps every 5 minutes so that you change resistance and wear on any specific joint area.

Recommendations for Various Budgets. When buying exercise equipment, you should be very careful how you spend your money. Often, after 2 or 3 weeks, the machine sits in a dusty corner in the basement and is not used. My choice for a year-round exercise machine is the mountain bicycle, which can be adapted to home use with a wind trainer for the back wheel. Many equipment decisions are dictated by budget concerns and financial matters. What follows is a list of buying recommendations for various budgetary categories.

$100 Budget (or Less)

- Select a series of 5- and 10-pound ankle weights that can be used for the upper and the lower body during walking and simple weight lifting.
- Purchase a used indoor exercise bicycle.

$500 Budget

- Select a series of free weights weighing from 5 to 10 pounds.
- Select a mountain bicycle at approximately $250 with a $125 wind trainer for year-round biking indoors and outdoors.
- Select a moderately priced ($100 or over) rowing machine for upper-body and back training.

$1,000 Budget

- In addition to 5- and 10-pound sandbags and a mountain bicycle, select an Aerodyne-type bicycle for upper- and lower-body exercise.

$3,000 Budget

- In addition to free weights, mountain bicycle, and wind trainer, select an indoor cross-country ski machine ($500) and a $1,000 electric treadmill.

Choosing Shoes

Shoes are undoubtedly the most important piece of equipment an athlete can buy; yet, for the serious runner and athlete, nothing is more confusing and frustrating than trying to find and buy shoes. Try to find a truly knowledgeable shoe salesperson who participates in your specific activity (running, soccer, dance, and so forth). Guidelines for choosing athletic shoes are actually very simple.

Avoid Testimonials. Most of us buy running shoes because of the hard sell from TV and magazine commercials with testimonials. The shoe industry is a multi-billion-dollar industry with high profits and high-paid testimonials, which are probably the least reliable source of information for the serious consumer. Very little scientific information is presented to help the consumer make an intelligent choice. Shoes have been promoted for their softness, air, gel, and shock absorption. However, the running companies have discovered that this is the best way to sell merchandise. Avoid the trap of buying a shoe simply because a world-class athlete uses it.

Avoid "Cheap Skates." The term *cheap skates* means exactly that. Inexpensive skates are bad for skating, and inexpensive shoes are bad for running and walking. One of your best protections is to buy the top-of-the-line model (in the range of $75 to $100 in 1990). Some of the manufacturers sell very expensive shoes to promote their name but also have very cheap models with a famous logo. Be careful of a cheap shoe with a fancy name.

Avoid "All Purpose" Shoe Companies. Some athletic shoe companies have hundreds of promotional items ranging from running bags and sports clothing to all types of athletic shoes. These companies' shoes include bedroom slippers, parachute shoes, boxing shoes, ice skates, basketball shoes, tennis shoes, and running shoes. If you are a runner, find an excellent running shoe that works for you. The same applies to other sports. Your coach, trainer, or physician can recommend a brand and type of shoe that will best meet your needs. (But, make sure that the coach is not being paid to endorse the shoe.)

Buy a Shoe That Fits. The first step in purchasing athletic shoes of any kind is deciding whether you will buy a straight "last" or a curved "last." The last is the sole of the shoe. A curved last encourages pronation, while a straight last resists it. Pronation is the lowering or the rolling-in motion of the inner, long arch of the foot, forming a flat foot. European shoes tend to be very narrow and straight, while American shoes tend to be somewhat wider and curved. In the early 1980s, many shoes had a curved last. Since then, studies have shown that during running the foot straightens and you should have more of a straight shoe. So, if your sport involves running, a straight shoe will be best.

If you are not sure what shape foot you have, try moving fast (run) while barefoot on a wet surface that will take an impression. If your footprint curves inward, then buy a curved-last shoe. If your footprint is straight, then buy a straight-last shoe. Look at your footprint while walking and while running. Generally, your walking footprint curves in, while the running footprint is straighter.

Buy a Shoe for Comfort and Protection. Many shoes now are marketed for shock absorption, but we have found that shock-absorption shoes are not stable enough and do not give you the protection and rear foot control needed for most sports activities. You should avoid shoes that are promoted for "performance" or "speed." It is highly unlikely that you will perform and run faster because of your shoe. You need a shoe for protection.

Choose a Shoe for the Right Features. The right features are these:

- **Forefoot Flexibility**—The normal foot flexes easily at the metatarsal region. Look at your foot and flex your toes and you will see where the forefoot creases. A good shoe will move like the normal foot. Inexpensive shoes or children's shoes are built on a board with very poor flexibility. Adults don't tolerate that rigid shoe and develop foot, ankle, and knee problems.
- **Torsional (Twisting) Stability**—Inexpensive shoes are either too rigid or too flexible when twisted. A good test is to take a running shoe and twist it as if you were squeezing a rag. It should resist the twisting and have good torsional stability for good control of your foot.
- **Firm Heel Control**—A sign of a poorly built shoe is a very flexible heel counter (the firm back area around the heel) with very poor support, such as what you would find in a bedroom slipper that has a soft heel and no counter. The more money you put into the shoe, the firmer the heel control becomes. This is a sign of a good shoe.

8. Nutrition

In December 1984, the National Institutes of Health made a strong statement recommending that Americans lower the fat and cholesterol content of their diets. Lifestyle guidelines for "Winning the Weighting Game" are provided in the appendix. It is recommended that the average athlete who is at an appropriate weight should maintain a diet that provides about 30 percent calories from fat.

For the overweight person with an elevated cholesterol level, a diet that provides 20 percent calories from fat is recommended. If you are overweight and active in a sport, you should establish a diet plan that adheres to the following guidelines:

- **Reduce Cholesterol**—When you think of cholesterol, think of meat and dairy products. Cholesterol is produced and found only in animal cells. Fish, meat, and dairy products are the primary direct sources of cholesterol, but it can be produced in humans when the dietary saturated fat content is increased. Athletes who watch their diets carefully should also be concerned about a cholesterol level that is too low. Athletes should keep their cholesterol levels below the 200-mg range.
- **Reduce Total Fat Content**—Fat is the highest source of calories in your diet with 9 calories per gram. Forty-five percent of calories in the typical Western diet comes from fat. This percentage should be significantly reduced, to 20 or 30 percent. The high fat content, whether it be from an animal or vegetable source, leads to elevated cholesterol, obesity, and cardiovascular disease.
- **Reduce Salt Intake**—The Western diet is saturated with salt to enhance flavor. The typical processed food items you purchase from the grocery store are full of salt. This added salt can contribute significantly to the development of cardiovascular disease. Since we automatically ingest a large quantity of salt from prepared foods, a first step in reducing salt intake is to avoid putting it on any foods.
- **Reduce Simple Sugar Intake**—White table sugar provides many extra calories but no nutritional value. Sugar is added to many foods for taste, but it only adds empty calories.
- **Increase Complex Carbohydrates**—By increasing carbohydrates, you will be providing energy and replacing your reduced intake of fats, sugar, meat, and dairy products.

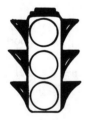

RED 45 percent of diet is fat calories—U.S. diet

YELLOW 30 percent of diet is fat calories—heart diet

GREEN 15-20 percent of diet is fat calories—low-fat diet

Serum Cholesterol and Activity

How activity affects cholesterol levels is of particular interest to the athlete. Our clinic conducted a study of 500 patients undergoing arthroscopic surgery. A serum blood cholesterol test was performed just prior to surgery. The study was published in the *American Medical Athletic Association Newsletter*, April 1988.

A positive correlation was found between those patients having chondromalacia (osteoarthritis) and elevated serum cholesterol. A serum cholesterol over 200 may be one of the risk factors associated with "wear and tear" of the joints. These preliminary findings may suggest that an elevated serum cholesterol may be a metabolic or vascular factor associated with the development of osteoarthritis.

The serum cholesterol test helps us differentiate between "healthy" and "fit" patients. The untimely death of marathon runner Jim Fixx reminds us that seemingly fit runners may not be as healthy as they appear. Fixx, who died unexpectedly following a run, had a cholesterol level of 250 mg. An autopsy revealed that besides extensive arteriosclerotic heart disease, he had an acute myocardial infarction.

We are unaware of other studies comparing various sports activities and serum cholesterol. Figure 2.1 notes the activities below and above the horizontal line, which is the serum cholesterol level of 200. Below 200 are the aerobic sports such as swimming, biking, running, tennis, and soccer. Above 200 are the large-muscled, nonaerobic sports such as football, skiing, and baseball. The highest cholesterol levels were found in bowlers.

Exercise obviously has an impact on cholesterol levels; however, activity does not "burn" cholesterol. Athletes who participate in aerobic sports such as

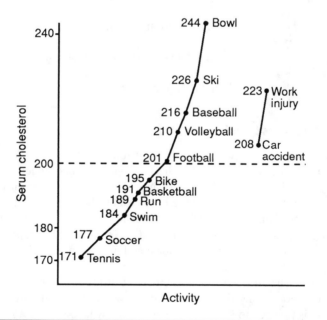

Figure 2.1 Activity vs. cholesterol. *Note.* From "Serum Cholesterol and Osteoarthritis" by G.N. Guten and D. Sheridan, 1988, *AMAA Newsletter*, **3**(2), p. 8. Copyright 1988 by American Medical Athletic Association. Reprinted by permission.

running, biking, and swimming have a lower cholesterol primarily because of genetic factors, metabolic lifestyle, and eating habits found in these performers. The second line on Figure 2.1 represents cholesterol levels of those in our practice with injuries not related to sports, including work- and accident-related injuries. This chart indicates that those people who were not active had higher cholesterol levels.

9. Fluids

Proper hydration (drinking enough water) is one of the few areas in sports medicine where listening to your body does not work. If you wait until you are thirsty, it is probably too late. You are already dehydrated. It is extremely important to drink early and plentifully during exercise. A helpful principle is ''a pint a pound, the world around,'' meaning that for every pound you lose, you must drink a pint of water (2 8-ounce glasses). It is beyond the scope of this book to discuss in depth the exercise physiology of dehydration and water needs. Suffice it to say that your cardiovascular system and your musculoskeletal system cannot work properly unless they have adequate fluid and electrolyte balance.

The red, yellow, and green classifications for fluids are as follows:

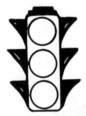

RED Avoid high salt, high sugar

YELLOW Low salt, low sugar, low caffeine

GREEN Water—best

Water: The Best Drink of All

The most important beverage to drink is water. There are two considerations when taking fluids, water and salt. The more poorly conditioned you are, the more salt you will lose. Therefore, early in your training, it is certainly advisable to add some salt to your fluids. There is no need to buy commercially prepared drinks that are costly and perhaps do not have the exact formula your body needs. Certain fluid supplements have alcohol and caffeine, which certainly give you a ''high'' but can also cause you to urinate and become more dehydrated as you urinate more. Water is the best drink.

Science so far has not developed the perfect drink for all athletes. The more you train, the more you will learn what drink will help you the most. The best advice again is to listen to your body to determine what beverage and how much is best. If you are interested in a drink other than water, a safe and moderate approach would be to purchase some of the commercially prepared drinks aimed at athletes and dilute them 25 to 50 percent. Don't be impressed by the commercials and endorsements, which can be misleading, exaggerated, and even untrue. In the final analysis, however, water is the key and is your best choice. Salt tablets should be avoided because they are too concentrated and tend to cause gastrointestinal upsets.

10. Surfaces

Of all treatment points, this may be the one most ignored by athletes. Yet the surface you hit has a major impact on your body. A surface can either discourage or encourage injuries. There are a wide range of possible surfaces for athletic competition; however, they can be divided into three basic types:

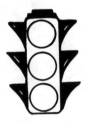

RED Avoid concrete

YELLOW Blacktop streets, indoor tracks (16 or fewer laps per mile)

GREEN Blacktop bicycle paths, or indoor paths (8–10 laps per mile)

Concrete and Wood

It is best to avoid these hard surfaces as much as possible. These surfaces don't "give" and thus can intensely jar the body on impact, resulting in serious injuries. Jokingly, a good rule of thumb is not to run on anything you wouldn't pound your head on.

Careful attention should be paid to surfaces for both high- and low-impact aerobics and other dancing activities. Suspended wood surfaces such as what ballerinas would choose are the best surfaces for these activities. You should avoid working out on carpeted surfaces with concrete underneath.

Blacktops, Bicycle Paths, Indoor Paths

For running and biking, blacktop bicycle paths are one of the best surfaces. Be very careful with indoor tracks that require more than 16 laps per mile. These will cause excessive twisting, turning, and stress to the ankle, knee, hip, and back.

It is beyond the scope of this book to compare football surfaces such as Astroturf and grass or tennis surfaces such as clay and grass. A general guideline is to find a surface that gives you the best traction and stability. A well-groomed surface probably gives you the best protection over artificial surfaces. Cost considerations and maintenance tend to lean toward the artificial surfaces, but these may have a higher incidence of twisting injuries.

Summary

The Stop, Caution, Go approach (using the red, yellow, and green classification system) for each of the points within the 10-Point Treatment Plan* are summarized below:

1. **Activity Levels**
   RED   Avoid hard use
   YELLOW   "Let pain be the guide"
   GREEN   Full use
               "Listen to your body"

2. **Alternative Activities** (twist or straight)
   RED   Avoid hard twist
               Basketball, volleyball, racquetball, wrestling
   YELLOW   Moderate twist
               Ski, dance, tennis, bowl, golf
   GREEN   Straight
               Walk, swim, bike, jog-run, cross-country ski, jump rope

3. **Rehab Exercises**
   RED   Avoid hard stretch
               Avoid vigorous bent joint with weights
   YELLOW   Moderate stretch
               Moderate bent joint with weights
   GREEN   Light stretch
               Joint straight—weights

4. **Support**
   RED   Cast
   YELLOW   Elastic sleeve, brace
   GREEN   Simple elastic wrap

5. **Thermal Treatment**
   RED   Avoid hot packs
   YELLOW   Lukewarm soaks
   GREEN   Ice packs

6. **Medication**
   RED   Avoid high dose vitamins
   YELLOW   Anti-inflammatory, ibuprofen
   GREEN   Aspirin, 2 per meal

---

*Note. The 10-Point Treatment Plan summary appeared in an earlier form in "A Ten-Point 'Stop and Go' Sports Medicine Program" by G.N. Guten, December 1986, *The Journal of Musculoskeletal Medicine*, pp. 24-26. Copyright 1986 by Cliggott Publishing Co. Adapted by permission.

7. **Equipment**
   RED   Avoid vigorous stair climbing
                     Avoid strenuous weight lifting
   YELLOW Rowing, trampoline
                     Moderate weight lifting
   GREEN   Treadmill, bike, cross-country ski

8. **Nutrition**—Food (percent of fat calories)
   RED   45 percent—U.S. diet
   YELLOW 30 percent—heart diet
   GREEN   15-20 percent—low-fat diet

9. **Fluids**
   RED   Avoid high salt, high sugar
   YELLOW Low salt, low sugar, low caffeine
   GREEN   Water—best

10. **Surfaces**
    RED   Avoid concrete
    YELLOW Blacktop streets
                      Indoor tracks 16/mile
    GREEN   Blacktop bike paths
                      Indoor tracks 8-10/mile

PART III

40 SPECIFIC INJURY TREATMENTS

You can locate a specific injury within Part III in four ways: (a) See the general head-to-toe organization by body part listed here; (b) see the following Anatomical Contents pages to find the appropriate pages; (c) use the section labels at the tops of pages; or (d) use the index at the end of this book.

The 40 specific treatment plans in Part III are organized by body parts in roughly a head-to-toe manner, as follows:

Each condition presents a specific 6-Point Condition Summary and a specific 10-Point Treatment Plan (see Part II for a general description). With this information, you can learn to listen to your body and establish the best activity level for your injury. All advice in Part III can be used after you have had a correct diagnosis of your problem from a health care professional. The specific rehabilitation exercise programs mentioned in each 10-Point Treatment plan can be found in Part IV.

Anatomical Contents

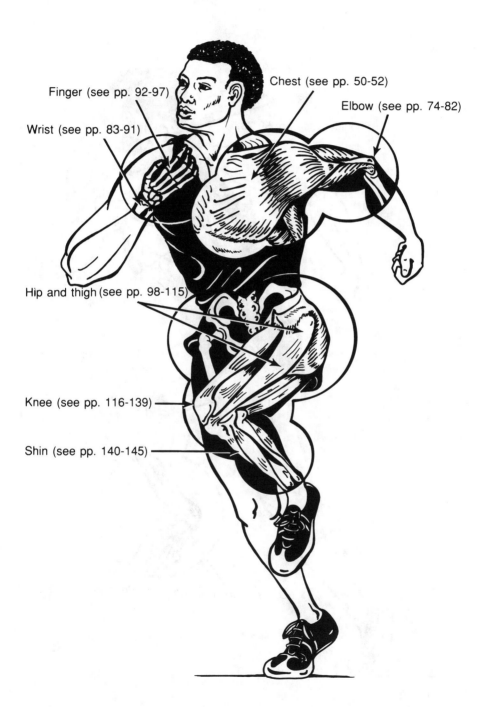

Finger (see pp. 92-97)

Chest (see pp. 50-52)

Elbow (see pp. 74-82)

Wrist (see pp. 83-91)

Hip and thigh (see pp. 98-115)

Knee (see pp. 116-139)

Shin (see pp. 140-145)

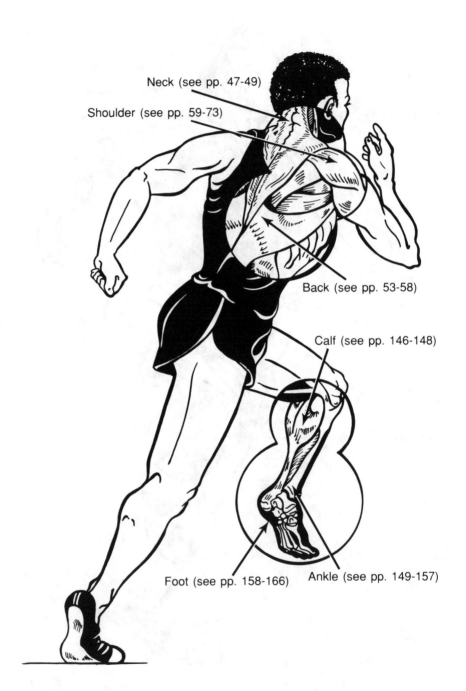

Neck (see pp. 47-49)

Shoulder (see pp. 59-73)

Back (see pp. 53-58)

Calf (see pp. 146-148)

Foot (see pp. 158-166)

Ankle (see pp. 149-157)

1. Herniated Disc

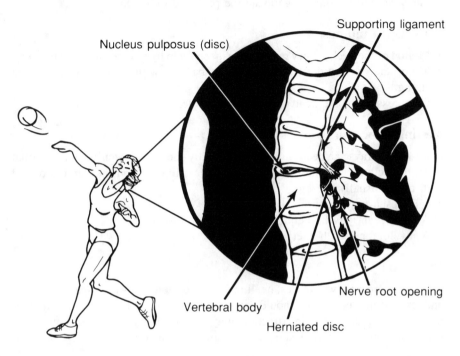

Supporting ligament

Nucleus pulposus (disc)

Nerve root opening

Vertebral body

Herniated disc

6-POINT CONDITION SUMMARY

Definition

A mechanical condition characterized by intense pain in the neck radiating down the arm, caused by nerve irritation from a disc degeneration, herniation, or bone spur.

Cause

- Acute local trauma to the neck.
- Chronic excessive twisting and hyperextension of the neck, causing undue pressure on the cervical disc and nerve root.

Subjective Symptoms

- Pain radiates from the back and side of the neck down to the shoulder, arm, and hand.
- Numbness or tingling radiates down the arm.
- Local swelling generally is not perceived.

- Stiffness in the neck exists, especially with extension and rotation.
- Sneezing and coughing aggravate the pain and radiation.

Objective Findings

- Motion of the neck is very restricted, especially in hyperextension and twisting.
- Motor and sensory deficits may exist in the arm, with reduced sensation and strength.
- Compression of the head and neck aggravates the pain.

Testing Procedures

- Routine X-rays can be normal but will usually show straightening of the normal cervical curvature. Narrowing and spur formation around the nerve root and discs are usually present.
- MRI tests may show disc herniation.
- A CAT scan may be helpful.
- A myelogram can be very diagnostic.

Prognosis

As with most nerve injuries, healing is very prolonged. Any impact, twisting, and extension maneuvers should be removed from athletic activity. If pain persists, hospitalization and traction may be necessary. Some patients need surgery to remove the discs and possibly fuse the spine for extreme degeneration.

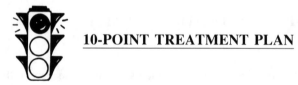 **10-POINT TREATMENT PLAN**

1. Activity Levels

- During periods of pain, avoid impact activities such as running.
- Walking, swimming, and biking may be satisfactory.
- If pain is caused by twisting of the neck while swimming, use a snorkel to breathe with the neck straight.

2. Alternative Activities

- Walking, swimming, and biking are excellent straight activities.
- As pain subsides, return to light twisting activities. Avoid impact.
- Use a mountain bicycle for biking so that you do not have to bend over and hyperextend the neck.

3. Rehab Exercises

- Do isometric exercises with local hand pressure to maintain muscle tone without moving the neck. As pain subsides, gradually increase motion and strength.
- See Back Flexion Program and Back Strengthening Program (these should be done only with the approval of your physician).

4. Support

- Use a simple wrap (like a towel) around the neck if a collar is not available. A semirigid collar may be of help during walking, running, and biking.

5. Thermal Treatment

- Use local heat to reduce muscle spasm.
- Local pain could be treated with ice massage.

6. Medication

- Simple anti-inflammatory medication is appropriate initially.
- If pain is very severe, codeine may be required.
- Avoid strong narcotics because of the chronic nature of the problem.
- Trigger point injections (at the site of muscle spasm) with steroid and Xylocaine sometimes help.

7. Equipment

- Use a hyperextension pad on football equipment to prevent the neck and head from overextending.

8. Nutrition

- Avoid obesity—follow a low-fat, high-carbohydrate diet.

9. Fluids

- Stay hydrated during training to maintain muscle function.

10. Surfaces

- Avoid jarring on hard surfaces such as hard roads and concrete.

2. Fracture of the Vertebra and Rib

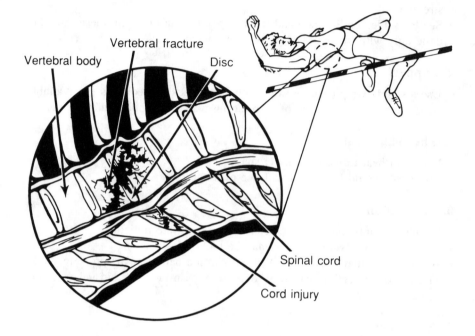

Vertebral fracture

Vertebral body

Disc

Spinal cord

Cord injury

6-POINT CONDITION SUMMARY

Definition

A traumatic condition associated with direct trauma to the bone of the thoracic vertebra or the adjacent rib structure.

Cause

- Compression (such as falling from a height) or a sudden jarring (such as bouncing in a toboggan) can cause thoracic spine injury.
- Rib fractures can occur from direct impact (as in football) or falling (as in skiing).

Subjective Symptoms

- Well-localized pain exists at the bony site.
- Local swelling may be present from the hematoma (collection of blood).
- Local stiffness occurs from spasm of the adjacent muscles.

Fracture of the Vertebra and Rib

- Coughing and sneezing are very painful.
- Nerve symptoms such as radiating pain and numbness may occur in the leg if the fracture is very severe and compresses the spinal cord.
- Coughing of blood and difficulty with breathing may occur if the rib injury seriously injures the lung.

Objective Findings

- Well-localized tenderness at the site of the bony injury.
- Difficulty with breathing due to possible lung injury by splinting and spasm of the adjacent muscle.
- Possible deficit of the nerves to the legs.

Testing Procedures

- Routine X-ray is very important for the rib, the lung, and the bone of the thoracic spine to find a bone injury or fluid in the lung.
- Initial X-rays could be negative if the fracture is minimal.
- Bone scan and MRI may be helpful in the first few days to pinpoint the fracture.

Prognosis

With no displacement of the fracture, healing is slow but progressive, with excellent results. Some thoracic fractures, if displaced, may require stabilization surgery, especially if there is spinal cord involvement. Rib fractures generally heal with minimal immobilization. In rare cases a rib fracture is serious and could puncture the lung and require immediate pulmonary management.

10-POINT TREATMENT PLAN

1. Activity Levels

- Rest is the initial activity, followed gradually by deep breathing, coughing, and gentle thoracic exercises during the first week.

2. Alternative Activities

- Nonimpact exercises are helpful—simple walking, swimming, and biking.
- Gradually progress within a week or two to light stationary biking followed by outdoor biking, depending on the type of fracture.
- Light jogging can be considered if there is no pain at 6–12 weeks. Let pain be the guide.

3. Rehab Exercises

- Rest is the treatment for the first several weeks.
- Gradually start deep breathing and mobilization exercises of the thoracic musculature.
- Begin simple push-ups and partial sit-ups as pain subsides.
- See Back Flexion Program and Back Strengthening Program (these should be done only with the approval of your physician).

4. Support

- A rib belt is very helpful.
- If the thoracic fracture is extensive, a fabricated metal or plastic hyperextension brace may be indicated.

5. Thermal Treatment

- Local ice to reduce swelling.
- Gradual use of heat to reduce muscle spasm.

6. Medication

- Simple anti-inflammatory medication such as aspirin or ibuprofen is appropriate.
- Stronger analgesics such as codeine may be required in the first few days because of bone pain.

7. Equipment

- A rib belt or a 6-inch elastic bandage wrapped around the thoracic spine is very helpful initially.
- More rigid thoracic supports may be in order if the fracture is severe.

8. Nutrition

- Because of rest and immobilization, obesity must be prevented.
- A low-fat, high-carbohydrate diet is best.

9. Fluids

- Maintain good hydration during periods of rest and training.

10. Surfaces

- Sleeping on a very firm mattress to control the spine is quite important. Training should be done on soft surfaces to avoid jarring.

3. Herniated or Slipped Disc

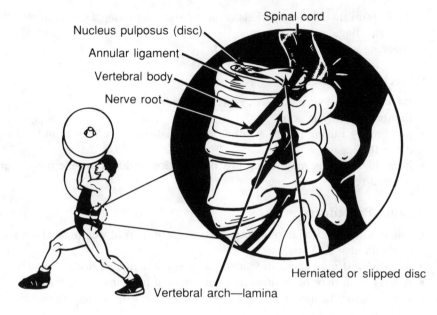

Spinal cord

Nucleus pulposus (disc)

Annular ligament

Vertebral body

Nerve root

Herniated or slipped disc

Vertebral arch—lamina

6-POINT CONDITION SUMMARY

Definition

A traumatic or degenerative condition characterized by localized breakdown or slipping of the nucleus pulposus (lumbar disc), causing direct inflammation and pressure on the lumbar nerve.

Cause

- Sudden exertion or extreme twisting, especially with the back in an extended position, causes a tear of the ligaments around the disc. This results in pressure and inflammation around the nerve root, leading to intense pain radiating down the back of the leg—"sciatica."
- In a middle-aged athlete (around the age of 40) the tissues are starting to "wear." A sudden twisting maneuver causes breakdown of the connective tissue, leading to direct inflammation of the nerve.

Subjective Symptoms

- Acute, sharp pain in the lumbar spine radiating into the hip and down to the leg.
- Numbness and tingling down the leg, aggravated by strain such as coughing or sitting.

Herniated or Slipped Disc

- Muscles guarded (tight) and spasmodic, especially with lumbar positions in extension.
- Pain aggravated by long periods of sitting such as driving a car. Pain relieved with standing.
- Sneezing and coughing very painful.

Objective Findings

- Back motion is very guarded, especially with extension.
- Lumbar stability is good.
- Straight-leg raising is very painful, with radiation of the pain from the back down the leg.
- Neurologic testing may reveal loss of sensation, reduced muscle power, and reduced reflexes.

Testing Procedures

- Initial X-rays may be normal or may show early signs of wearing and thinning of the lumbar disc spaces.
- An MRI test may be positive and may show a herniated disc.
- A CAT scan may be positive and may show a lumbar disc herniation.
- A myelogram (a specialized dye test) of the lumbar spine may show the disc pressing on a nerve.
- EMG nerve testing after several weeks may show the nerve injury.

Prognosis

Healing can be very slow because of the nerve injury. Hospitalization and traction may be required if bed rest at home does not help after 1 or 2 weeks. Surgery may be necessary if pain persists or increasing neurologic deficits develop after several weeks.

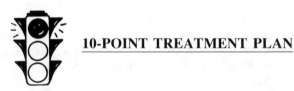

10-POINT TREATMENT PLAN

1. Activity Levels

- Avoid any exercise that includes impact, twisting, or bending; err on the side of overresting.
- As pain subsides, start to walk, then swim, and then bike.
- Avoid activities that include impact for at least 6 weeks.

2. Alternative Activities

- Use a stationary bicycle and swim during the initial weeks of rehabilitation.

- Avoid anything that will hyperextend and twist the spine.
- Run in a swimming pool with a Wet Vest.

3. Rehab Exercises

- Rest is indicated, especially with the knees bent.
- Deep breathing and gentle leg and arm motion are helpful during early periods of pain.
- During periods of rehabilitation, do sit-ups and flexion exercises to maintain abdominal strength.
- See Back Flexion Program and Back Strengthening Program (should be done only with the approval of your physician).

4. Support

- Various lumbar braces can be tried but should not be a substitute for bed rest and good judgment.

5. Thermal Treatment

- Because of the muscle spasm, initial heat is best for muscle relaxation.
- Heat is most effective for the large muscle groups. Switch to ice when the pain becomes very pinpoint.

6. Medication

- Take simple anti-inflammatory medication such as ibuprofen.
- Muscle relaxers may be indicated but can cause excessive sleepiness.
- If pain persists, a steroid injection directly around the nerve root, called an "epidural" injection, may be done.

7. Equipment

- Lie on a very firm surface such as the floor or a very hard bed.

8. Nutrition

- Because of the bed rest, avoid overeating.
- A low-fat, high-carbohydrate diet is best.
- Don't overeat during periods of frustration and depression.

9. Fluids

- Maintain good hydration during periods of rest and training to maintain muscle function and urinary flow.

10. Surfaces

- Avoid hills and hard surfaces during rehabilitation.
- Stay on blacktop and bicycle paths for exercise.
- Sleep on very firm surfaces.

4. Muscle Tear

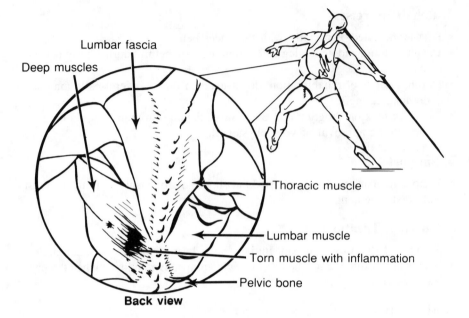

Lumbar fascia

Deep muscles

Thoracic muscle

Lumbar muscle

Torn muscle with inflammation

Pelvic bone

Back view

6-POINT CONDITION SUMMARY

Definition

A traumatic condition characterized by a localized tearing of the muscle of the low back, causing local pain, spasm, and occasional radiation of discomfort.

Cause

- Localized muscle tearing due to a rapid twisting maneuver, generally with the spine in either extreme flexion or extension.
- Injuries such as bruising from direct impact such as in football.

Subjective Symptoms

- Well-localized pain in the low back area with occasional radiation into the hip and groin.
- Tightness of muscle, especially with bending. Pain aggravated by sneezing, coughing, and sitting.
- Neurologic symptoms such as numbness or intense radiation down the leg generally not present.

Objective Findings

- Motion of the lumbar spine is restricted, especially in flexion or extension.
- Stability of the spine is good.
- Muscles are generally tight, but there is no swelling. Neurologic exam is negative.

Testing Procedures

- Routine X-rays are generally normal.
- Neurologic exam and special nerve tests are negative.
- MRI is generally not helpful, unless severe soft-tissue muscle injury is present.

Prognosis

Healing potential is good but can be very prolonged, taking weeks to months. Some cases require hospitalization, traction, and prolonged bed rest if the muscle injury is serious. Surgery is not indicated, unless a herniated disc is associated.

 10-POINT TREATMENT PLAN

1. Activity Levels

- Keep knees bent during the period of rest (on a bed or a semireclining chair).
- Straight activities such as walking, swimming, and biking are best at the beginning of recovery.

2. Alternative Activities

- Use a stationary bicycle and swim during the initial weeks of rehabilitation.
- Avoid anything that will hyperextend and twist the spine.
- Run in a swimming pool with a Wet Vest.

3. Rehab Exercises

- First, rest in bed, keeping the knees bent.
- As pain subsides within a few days to a week, begin gentle flexion and extension exercises such as sit-ups, push-ups, and swimming.
- See Back Flexion Program and Back Strengthening Program (these should be done only with the approval of your physician).

4. Support

- Various lumbar supports are available.
- Wrap several elastic wraps around the lumbar spine.
- Initially, taping can be used.
- Lumbar corsets are available to help protect the spine during early sports activities.

5. Thermal Treatment

- Use local ice massage to reduce spasm.
- If large muscle groups are involved, heat can be tried before ice for muscle relaxation.

6. Medication

- Use simple anti-inflammatory medications such as aspirin and ibuprofen.
- Try muscle relaxers. Generally they will cause excessive sleepiness.
- Sometimes a local steroid injection may be indicated in the inflamed muscle after several weeks of rehabilitation.

7. Equipment

- Wrap the lumbar spine with elastic wraps or corset to protect the back.

8. Nutrition

- Avoid obesity, especially because of periods of reduced activity.
- Avoid eating out of "frustration." A low-fat, high-carbohydrate diet is best.

9. Fluids

- Maintain good hydration during periods of rest and training to maintain muscle function.

10. Surfaces

- Avoid hills, which will aggravate the lumbar strain.
- Use flat, soft surfaces such as blacktops and bicycle paths for early exercise routines.
- Sleep on very firm surfaces.

5. Acromioclavicular Joint (AC) Separation

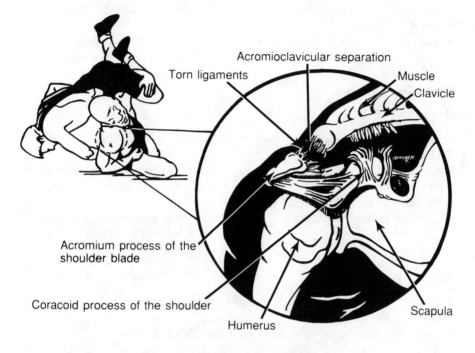

Acromioclavicular separation

Torn ligaments

Muscle

Clavicle

Acromium process of the shoulder blade

Coracoid process of the shoulder

Humerus

Scapula

6-POINT CONDITION SUMMARY

Definition

A traumatic displacement and separation at the end of the collar bone (clavicle) from the tip of the shoulder (acromion) due to violent tearing of the ligaments that stabilize the clavicle. There are three grades:

Grade I—Minimal displacement
Grade II—Moderate displacement
Grade III—Severe displacement (may require surgery)

Cause

- Direct fall on the side of the shoulder.
- Indirect fall on an outstretched arm, causing the clavicle to displace due to torn ligaments.

Acromioclavicular Joint (AC) Separation

Subjective Symptoms

Acute

- Sudden pain at the top of the shoulder following a fall.
- Local swelling.
- Inability to lift the arm overhead.

Chronic

- Ache with use.
- Grinding sensation with shoulder use.
- Pain with overhead sports activities such as throwing.

Objective Findings

Acute

- Well-localized tenderness at the tip of the clavicle at the AC joint.
- Local swelling.
- Local deformity.
- Negative neurovascular test.
- Shoulder motion restricted.

Chronic

- A small spur or bump may be palpated at the AC joint.
- Local swelling may be present.
- Crepitation or noise can be heard or felt.
- Motion is almost normal but may be restricted on extreme overhead motion.

Testing Procedures

- Routine X-rays vary, revealing minimal displacement in Grade I to extreme displacement in Grade III.
- Bone scan may be positive for bone inflammation in chronic cases.
- In rare cases an MRI test may be helpful for showing tear of the ligaments and the meniscus of the joint.

Prognosis

Healing is generally very satisfactory in Grade I and Grade II cases. Grade III cases may be left with a painful bump and deformity on the tip of the shoulder. In most cases, this bump and deformity do not limit function but may be associated with moderate weakness. Some surgeons will recommend surgical repair in Grade III cases to restore the anatomy in high performance athletes.

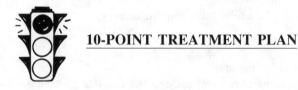

10-POINT TREATMENT PLAN

1. Activity Levels

- Immobilization of the shoulder with a sling for Grade I and Grade II tears. Grade III tears may require surgery or a special harness.

Acromioclavicular Joint (AC) Separation

2. Alternative Activities

- The patient may walk and lightly jog and bicycle.
- Running in a swimming pool with a Wet Vest is permitted, but arm motion is not permitted.

3. Rehab Exercises

- Do isometric tightening exercises to maintain muscle tone during initial period of immobilization and sling.
- Gradually increase muscle flexibility, endurance, speed, and strength with gentle weight lifting as the sling becomes unnecessary.
- See Beginning Shoulder Program. Progress to Shoulder Acromioclavicular Program.

4. Support

- First aid in sling and elastic wraps.
- Special harness for acromioclavicular joint in selected cases.

5. Thermal Treatment

- Local ice to reduce pain and inflammation for the first 1 to 2 days.
- Local heat to reduce muscle spasm after the first few days.

6. Medication

- During acute phase, codeine and Demerol may be needed in the first 1 to 2 days.
- For chronic pain, simple aspirin and nonsteroidal medication may be required.
- After several months of local pain and inflammation, a local steroid injection may be indicated.

7. Equipment

- During periods of immobilization, leg exercises and biking are permissible.

8. Nutrition

- Avoid fluids or food for the first several hours after injury because of the rare possibility of open surgery.
- Maintain a high-carbohydrate, low-fat diet.

9. Fluids

- Maintain fluid intake and good hydration after surgery has been performed or ruled out.

10. Surfaces

- Use nonskid running surfaces to avoid falls on the arm.

6. Anterior Dislocation

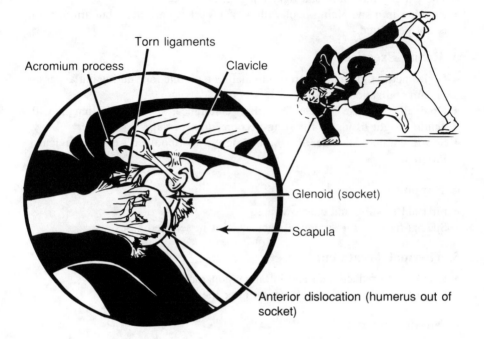

Torn ligaments

Acromium process

Clavicle

Glenoid (socket)

Scapula

Anterior dislocation (humerus out of socket)

6-POINT CONDITION SUMMARY

Definition

A traumatic condition in which the ball of the shoulder (humerus) completely separates from the socket (glenoid). The displacement is usually forward (anterior).

Cause

- Direct trauma to the side of the shoulder during a fall on the shoulder.
- Indirect shoulder trauma by fall on the outstretched hand.
- Congenital looseness (laxity) of the joint due to bony abnormality or ligament insufficiency.

Subjective Symptoms

- Acute, intense pain on the front of the shoulder.
- Local swelling and a mass perceived (the humerus bone).
- Inability to move the arm.
- Occasional numbness in the hand, if nerve pressure is present.

Objective Findings

- Arm rotated outward.
- Inability to move the arm due to pain, weakness, and deformity.
- Bony mass felt on the front of the shoulder.
- Nerve exam usually normal, but nerve damage present in some cases.

Testing Procedures

- X-ray will show displacement of the head of the humerus. Associated fracture may be present.
- Bone scan and MRI are not needed in early cases but may be helpful in chronic recurrent cases.
- EMG may show nerve impingement.

Prognosis

Most cases heal if proper rest and immobilization is done in the acute case. Teenage patients have a higher rate of recurrence. Immediate closed reduction after an X-ray is required. Often this is done with a local or general anesthetic. Some cases develop ''recurrent dislocation,'' which may require surgical stabilization. Certain rotation motions may have to be avoided. The return to sports is often delayed several months until flexibility, endurance, speed, and strength are improved.

10-POINT TREATMENT PLAN

1. Activity Levels

- Complete immobilization of the shoulder for several weeks to allow healing of the injured muscles and ligaments.
- Then a gradual program of pendulum swinging of the arm to full-motion exercises.

2. Alternative Activities

- Walking, stationary biking, and light jogging are permitted if pain is minimal and there is no jarring.

3. Rehab Exercises

- During sling immobilization of the first month, do isometric tightening of the shoulder and neck muscles.

- Once sling is removed, start exercises to build flexibility, endurance, speed, and strength by using tubing and free weights.
- See Beginning Shoulder Program for early rehabilitation. Progress to Shoulder Dislocation Program for later rehabilitation.

4. Support

- Acute phase: First aid in a sling or wrapping the shoulder with an elastic bandage.
- Post reduction: sling and shoulder wrap.
- Rehabilitation: simple collar and cuff to allow pendulum exercises and gradual mobilization.

5. Thermal Treatment

- Local ice to the shoulder for the first 1 to 2 days to reduce pain and swelling.
- Local heat to reduce muscle spasm after 1 to 2 days.

6. Medication

- Acute pain is treated with codeine and possibly a Demerol injection for the closed reduction.
- During rehabilitation, simple aspirin or anti-inflammatory medication should be taken.
- A local steroid injection sometimes is required for scarring and inflammation several months after rehabilitation.

7. Equipment

- A special shoulder harness may be used for sports to prevent external rotation and recurrent dislocation.

8. Nutrition

- Avoid obesity during period of immobilization; eat a high-carbohydrate, low-fat diet.

9. Fluids

- Immediately after the injury the patient should drink nothing by mouth because of the possibility of closed reduction under general anesthesia.

10. Surfaces

- Light running and twisting sports may be done on nonskid surfaces so that the patient does not slip and injure the arm again.

7. Rotator Cuff Tendinitis and Tear

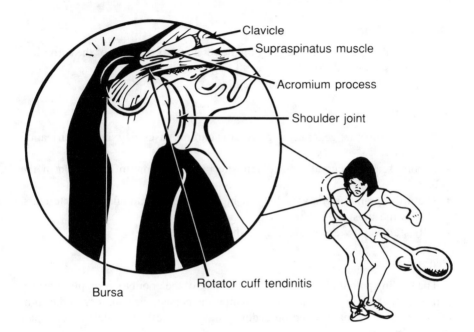

Clavicle

Supraspinatus muscle

Acromium process

Shoulder joint

Bursa

Rotator cuff tendinitis

6-POINT CONDITION SUMMARY

Definition

A local overuse inflammation to the group of four major shoulder muscles that run together, attach to the humerus, and form a heavy tendon called the "rotator cuff." Overhead activities may impinge the cuff and cause wear and tear.

Cause

- Repetitive overhead activities such as throwing or playing tennis with the shoulder at 90 degrees will stretch and impinge the cuff, causing local wear and tear.
- Acute symptoms may occur in a sudden fall.

Subjective Symptoms

- Pain well localized to the anterior lateral aspect of the shoulder just below the acromion. The symptoms may radiate around the shoulder or down the arm.
- Stiffness and difficulty with overhead activities.

- Weakness, a common major complaint, especially difficulty in pulling the arm away from the body (abduction).
- Crepitation, grinding sensation with motion.
- Night pain common.

Objective Findings

- Well-localized tenderness directly on the rotator cuff at the tip of the acromion.
- Weakness, especially with arm at 90 degrees.
- Crepitation sometimes heard and felt.

Testing Procedures

- Regular X-rays are generally negative, but chronic cases may show calcification or spurs.
- A bone scan is generally not diagnostic but may show inflammation of the bone.
- The arthrogram can be very helpful in large incomplete and complete tears. This is the most diagnostic.
- MRI studies now are beginning to show early tears.

Prognosis

The healing potential is not excellent because of the poor blood supply. Restrict activities that cause the condition. If symptoms persist, then surgery in the form of arthroscopy or major open procedures may be necessary to debride or repair the tendon.

10-POINT TREATMENT PLAN

1. Activity Levels

- Restrict extreme overhead activities.
- Modify throwing, tennis, and biking maneuvers to keep the shoulder below 90 degrees.

2. Alternative Activities

- Avoid twisting and torqueing activities.
- Work more on biking, swimming, and running.
- Gradually increase throwing in a moderate program.

Rotator Cuff Tendinitis and Tear

3. Rehab Exercises

- Progressive stiffness must be prevented.
- Flexibility and strengthening exercises are very important.
- See Beginning Shoulder Program. Progress to Rotator Cuff Program.

4. Support

- Braces are generally not effective, but gentle wrapping of the shoulder with an elastic wrap sometimes will help during acute pain.

5. Thermal Treatment

- Local ice to reduce inflammation of the surrounding tendon and bursa.
- Local heat to relax and mobilize the tight shoulder muscles.

6. Medication

- Start with simple analgesics and anti-inflammatory medication.
- Progress to local steroid injection before considering surgery.

7. Equipment

- Proper selection of tennis rackets, baseball bats, and throwing apparatus is very important.
- Choose equipment that has minimal vibration.

8. Nutrition

- Maintain low body fat with a high-carbohydrate, low-fat diet.

9. Fluids

- Maintain good hydration with good fluid intake.

10. Surfaces

- Minimize jarring by avoiding running on concrete and excessively banked or curved hills.

8. Rupture of Biceps Tendon

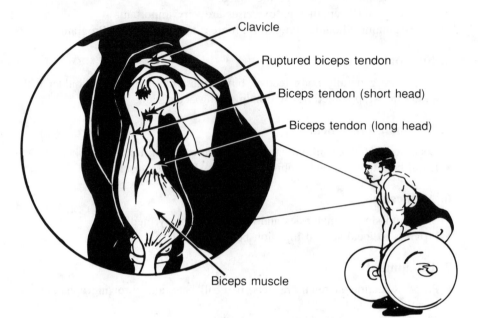

Clavicle

Ruptured biceps tendon

Biceps tendon (short head)

Biceps tendon (long head)

Biceps muscle

6-POINT CONDITION SUMMARY

Definition

A traumatic overuse condition resulting in a sudden tearing of the biceps tendon in the front of the shoulder.

Cause

- Violent, heavy lifting that overloads the tendon, resulting in tearing.
- Repetitive, overhead lifting, generally in a middle-aged athlete.

Subjective Symptoms

- Acute pain and perception of a "pop" on the front of the shoulder.
- Sudden weakness with lifting.
- Muscle mass perceived and felt in the front of the mid-arm.

Objective Findings

- Local tenderness directly on the front of the shoulder, 2 to 3 inches below the clavicle.

- Local swelling possible with bruising.
- Weakness of flexor muscle group.
- Nerve function intact.

Testing Procedures

- X-rays generally are not helpful, but a spur may be present.
- Bone scan and MRI are generally not required to make the diagnosis.
- Arthroscopy is rarely indicated.

Prognosis

Surgery is rarely indicated. Weakness is rarely a problem after adequate rehabilitation. Healing generally accomplished without surgery.

10-POINT TREATMENT PLAN

1. Activity Levels

- Let pain be the guide for the first month.
- No lifting is allowed during the first month but isometric exercises are permitted to maintain muscle tone.

2. Alternative Activities

- Running, biking, swimming, and running in a swimming pool are all permitted.

3. Rehab Exercises

- Light flexion exercises during the acute phase.
- Shoulder rehabilitation exercises with tubing and sandbags.
- See Beginning Shoulder Program. Progress to Shoulder Acromioclavicular Program.

4. Support

- Sling for 1 to 2 weeks.

5. Thermal Treatment

- Local ice for the initial 1 to 2 days for pain and swelling.
- Local heat after a few days for muscle spasm.

6. Medication

- In the first 1 to 2 days, codeine may be required, followed by aspirin or nonsteroidal anti-inflammatory medication.
- If chronic pain persists after several months, a local steroid injection may be indicated.

7. Equipment

- Modification of intense weight-lifting equipment to simple free weights, and select tennis rackets that dampen the vibration (reduce string tension).

8. Nutrition

- Avoid obesity with a high-carbohydrate, low-fat diet.

9. Fluids

- Maintain good hydration during periods of training to maintain muscle function.

10. Surfaces

- A nonskid surface should be used to avoid any further falls on an outstretched arm.

9. Subacromial Bursitis

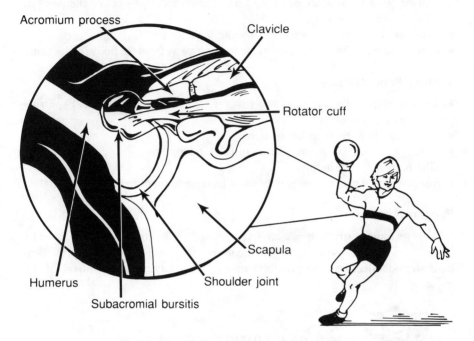

Acromium process

Clavicle

Rotator cuff

Scapula

Shoulder joint

Humerus

Subacromial bursitis

6-POINT CONDITION SUMMARY

Definition

A traumatic overuse condition characterized by local pain and stiffness due to inflammation in the bursa and tendon between the bones of the shoulder.

Cause

- Repetitive overhead arm use such as throwing or playing tennis.
- Direct trauma or fall on the side of the shoulder.
- Early tear of the rotator cuff, resulting in inflammation of the bursa.

Subjective Symptoms

- Pain with shoulder use, usually overhead.
- Noise and crepitation with shoulder use.
- Swelling usually not present.
- Stiffness moderate.

Objective Findings

- Tenderness is well localized to the tip of the shoulder just below the point of the shoulder (acromion).
- Swelling is usually not perceived by the physician.
- There is pain and limitation of moving the arm away from the body (abduction).

Testing Procedures

- X-ray is usually negative in early cases. Late cases may show local spurring and degenerative changes.
- Scan may show bone inflammation.
- Arthrogram may show small tears in the tendon.
- MRI is usually not helpful.
- Arthroscopy in chronic cases may show inflammation of the bursa and tendon.

Prognosis

With rest and restriction of activity, pain and inflammation usually subside. Some cases require more aggressive treatment with anti-inflammatory medication, steroid injection, and possibly arthroscopic shaving and removal of the bursa.

 10-POINT TREATMENT PLAN

1. Activity Levels

- Let pain be the guide.
- Minimize overhead activities.

2. Alternative Activities

- Running, biking, swimming, and use of a Wet Vest are permitted.
- Restrict racket sports to forehand and not overhead strokes.

3. Rehab Exercises

- Avoid overhead abduction.
- Use gentle pendulum range of motion to loosen the shoulder and progressively use tubing and sandbags to maintain flexibility, endurance, speed, and strength.
- See Beginning Shoulder Program. Progress to Rotator Cuff Program.

4. Support

- Braces and slings are generally not helpful.

5. Thermal Treatment

- Local ice massage after pain or after exercise workout.
- Heat before athletic use to relax muscles.

6. Medication

- Moderate pain treated with aspirin and nonsteroidal anti-inflammatory medication.
- Local steroid injection sometimes very helpful.

7. Equipment

- Isokinetic exercises of the upper shoulder to maintain shoulder strength.
- Aerodyne bicycle for arm and leg use.
- Tennis racket changes to reduce vibration and torqueing. Choose a racket with a thick hand grip, a wide face, and reduced string tension.

8. Fluids

- Maintain good hydration during periods of training to maintain muscle function and urine flow.

9. Nutrition

- Maintain body weight with a high-carbohydrate, low-fat diet.

10. Surfaces

- Play on nonskid racket surfaces to avoid falling on an outstretched arm.

10. Lateral Epicondylitis (Tennis Elbow)

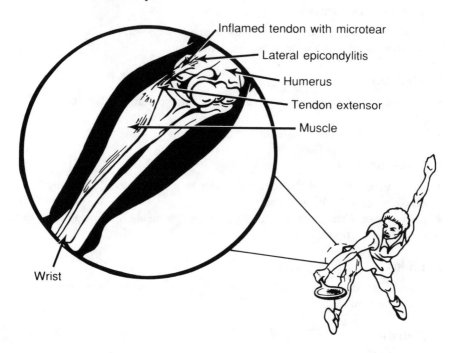

Inflamed tendon with microtear
Lateral epicondylitis
Humerus
Tendon extensor
Muscle
Wrist

6-POINT CONDITION SUMMARY

Definition

A local inflammation on the outer (lateral) side of the elbow at the lateral epicondyle, due to repeated microtrauma resulting in local elbow pain.

Cause

- Acute, sudden, violent injury and tearing of the muscle can cause an acute tennis elbow.
- Chronic, repeated strain and pulling of the extensor forearm muscles in racket or club sports activities such as the backhand swing of tennis, or excessive swing with the left arm in a right-handed golfer, can cause tennis elbow.

Subjective Symptoms

- Pain is well localized to the outer (lateral) side of the elbow. The pain may radiate down the forearm.

Lateral Epicondylitis (Tennis Elbow)

- Swelling is generally not present.
- Stiffness may be present but is generally not a feature.
- Pain is aggravated by wrist activities such as lifting a coffee pot or a heavy object with the palm down (pronated).

Objective Findings

- Tenderness well localized to the muscle attachment to the side of the elbow.
- Weakness of the wrist extensor group due to pain and inflammation.
- Loss of motion not present.

Testing Procedures

- Routine X-rays are generally negative, but a small spur may be present in the elbow.
- Bone scan may be of help in showing local inflammation.
- EMG studies are usually negative.
- MRI studies are generally not helpful.

Prognosis

Healing in the tendon can be prolonged because of poor blood supply to the tendon. After months of conservative treatment for inflammation, surgery may be necessary to remove offending scar tissue.

 ## 10-POINT TREATMENT PLAN

1. Activity Levels

- Continue to play moderate tennis and racquet sports, but avoid backhand maneuvers.

2. Alternative Activities

- Running, biking, and swimming are very helpful for maintaining aerobic exercise.

3. Rehab Exercises

- Maintain a balance of exercises to develop flexibility and strength, especially in the wrist extensor muscle group.
- See Upper Extremity Stretching Program. Progress to Beginning Tennis Elbow Program and Advanced Tennis Elbow Program, using manual resistance and tubing.

Lateral Epicondylitis (Tennis Elbow)

4. Support

- A tennis elbow band, worn 1 or 2 inches below the elbow, helps compress and immobilize the muscle group.

5. Thermal Treatment

- Local ice massage is very helpful.
- Use heat to mobilize muscles.

6. Medication

- Start with simple analgesics and anti-inflammatory medication.
- Progress to local steroid injection before considering surgery.

7. Equipment

- Tennis rackets that dampen the vibration are very important.
- Choose equipment that has thick hand grips and rackets that are wide bodied.
- Reduce string tension in rackets.

8. Nutrition

- Maintain low body fat with a high-carbohydrate, low-fat diet.

9. Fluids

- Maintain good hydration with good fluid intake.

10. Surfaces

- Run on bike paths (asphalt is best). Avoid running on concrete, which will further jar the body.
- Play tennis on cushioned surfaces, but be careful of twisting activities.

11. Medial Epicondylitis (Baseball Elbow)

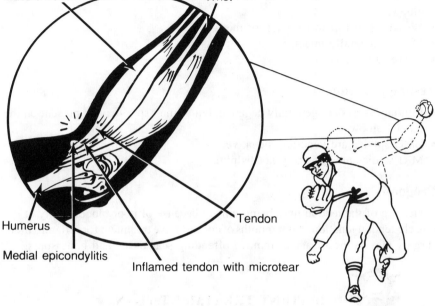

Muscle flexor Wrist

Humerus

Medial epicondylitis

Inflamed tendon with microtear

Tendon

6-POINT CONDITION SUMMARY

Definition

A local traumatic condition on the inner (medial) aspect of the elbow at the medial epicondyle, due to repetitive microtrauma, throwing, or twisting.

Cause

- Acute, sudden throwing injury due to violent twisting of the elbow.
- Chronic, repetitive strain and pulling of the flexor forearm muscles from throwing curve balls, hitting a golf ball, or doing the twist serve in tennis.

Subjective Symptoms

- Pain well localized at the inner aspect of the elbow, with pain radiating to the inner forearm.
- Swelling generally not present.
- Stiffness may be present but generally not a feature.

Medial Epicondylitis (Baseball Elbow)

- Pain aggravated by lifting objects with the palm up (supinated).
- Numbness not a feature, unless there is ulnar nerve involvement.

Objective Findings

- Tenderness well localized at the muscle attachment to the inner side of the elbow.
- Weakness in forearm flexion of the wrist.
- Motion generally intact.
- Nerve exam negative.

Testing Procedures

- Routine X-rays are generally negative, but a small spur may be present on the medial elbow.
- EMG studies are generally negative.
- MRI studies are generally not helpful.

Prognosis

Healing of the tendon may be prolonged because of poor blood supply at the muscle-tendon junction. After months of conservative treatment for inflammation, surgery may be necessary to remove offending scar tissue and bone spurs.

10-POINT TREATMENT PLAN

1. Activity Levels

- Continue to play moderate tennis and racket sports, but avoid excessive forehand maneuvers.

2. Alternative Activities

- Running, biking, and swimming are all very helpful for maintaining aerobic exercise.

3. Rehab Exercises

- Maintain a balance of exercises to develop flexibility and strength, especially in the wrist flexor muscle group.
- See Upper Extremity Stretching Program. Progress to Beginning Tennis Elbow Program and to Advanced Tennis Elbow Program, using manual resistance and tubing.

Medial Epicondylitis (Baseball Elbow)

4. Support

- A tennis elbow band is not as helpful as it is on the lateral side of the elbow.

5. Thermal Treatment

- Local ice massage is very helpful for reducing inflammation.
- Use heat to mobilize muscles before activity.

6. Medication

- Start with simple analgesics and anti-inflammatory medication.
- Progress to local steroid injection before considering surgery.

7. Equipment

- Proper tennis rackets with thick hand grips will dampen vibration.

8. Nutrition

- Maintain low body fat with a high-carbohydrate, low-fat diet.

9. Fluids

- Maintain proper hydration with good fluid intake.

10. Surfaces

- Run on bike paths (asphalt is best). Avoid running on concrete, which may further jar the body.
- Play tennis on cushioned surfaces, but be careful of twisting activities.

12. Ulnar Nerve Entrapment

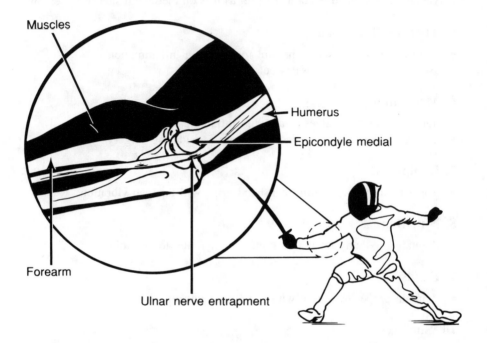

Muscles

Humerus

Epicondyle medial

Forearm

Ulnar nerve entrapment

6-POINT CONDITION SUMMARY

Definition

A local traumatic condition to the inner (medial) elbow, causing acute or chronic nerve symptoms with pain and numbness.

Cause

- Acute injury to the inner (medial) elbow at the "crazy bone," the ulnar nerve.
- Chronic overuse in throwing or golfing, of a malaligned elbow, causing stretching of the ulnar nerve.

Subjective Symptoms

- Pain at the elbow, radiating to the fourth and fifth fingers (ulnar nerve distribution).
- Numbness of the forearm, radiating to the fourth and fifth fingers.
- Weakness of fingers in severe cases.

Objective Findings

- Tenderness well localized to the inner elbow, directly on the ulnar nerve in the groove.
- Numbness and weakness of the hand.
- Motion intact.

Testing Procedures

- X-rays are generally negative, but a small spur may be present on the inner elbow.
- Bone scan and MRI are generally not helpful.
- EMG test may show chronic changes in the ulnar nerve.

Prognosis

Slow healing is generally possible with rest and by avoiding strenuous activities. Some chronic cases may need transfer and decompression of the nerve by surgical techniques.

 10-POINT TREATMENT PLAN

1. Activity Levels

- Minimize overhead throwing and any activity that can torque the elbow.

2. Alternative Activities

- Aerobic sports such as running, biking, and swimming are permitted.

3. Rehab Exercises

- Maintain range of motion and develop flexibility and strength with sandbags and tubing.
- See Upper Extremity Stretching Program. Progress to Beginning Tennis Elbow Program and Advanced Tennis Elbow Program, using manual resistance and tubing.
- Avoid excessive stretching or any symptoms that cause nerve symptoms.

4. Support

- Avoid any compressive, tight bandages around the elbow.
- Use foam pads to protect elbow.

5. Thermal Treatment

- Local ice massage to reduce nerve inflammation.
- Heat to be used before activities for muscle relaxation.

6. Medication

- Anti-inflammatory medication is sometimes helpful for reducing nerve inflammation. Some physicians recommend multivitamins for nerve regeneration.
- Local steroid injection is sometimes helpful for reducing inflammation.

7. Equipment

- Use tennis racket with a large grip.

8. Nutrition

- Maintain a high-carbohydrate, low-fat diet.

9. Fluids

- Maintain proper hydration with good fluid intake.

10. Surfaces

- Avoid running on hard surfaces to minimize jarring.
- Play tennis on cushioned surfaces, but be careful of any twisting activities or falls.
- Do not rest the elbow on the side of a chair or a desk.

13. Carpal Tunnel

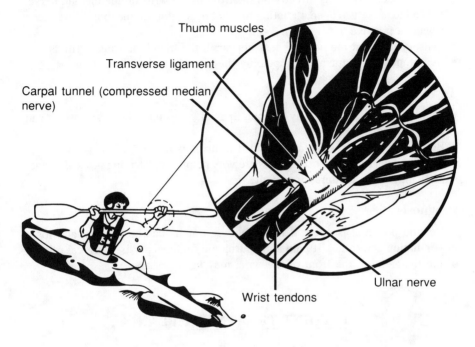

Thumb muscles

Transverse ligament

Carpal tunnel (compressed median nerve)

Ulnar nerve

Wrist tendons

6-POINT CONDITION SUMMARY

Definition

A local inflammation characterized by pressure on or about the median nerve at the wrist, resulting in pain and numbness, especially when the wrist is in a flexed position.

Cause

- An acute injury, such as local trauma or compression, to the front (anterior) aspect of the wrist, causing local pain and swelling.
- A chronic, repetitive, bent-wrist activity such as typing, manual labor, or sleeping in a flexed position.

Subjective Symptoms

- Pain exists, especially in the radiation of the median nerve along the first three fingers and thumb, and especially at night.
- Strength may become reduced, especially in pinching.
- The wrist feels less pain when it is in an extended neutral position rather than a flexed position.

Objective Findings

- Local tenderness exists directly on the front of the wrist on the median nerve. When the nerve is tapped, radiating numbness develops in the thumb and index finger (a positive Tinel sign).
- Sensory loss and motor weakness appear in the thumb and index finger.
- Symptoms are aggravated by placing the wrist in a flexed position.

Testing Procedures

- Routine X-rays are generally normal. Special views may show a small spur in the wrist.
- Bone scan may show inflammation if arthritis is present.
- EMG and nerve conduction studies are very helpful in detecting nerve damage.
- MRI may show compression of the nerve.

Prognosis

Healing potential is good, if the offending trauma can be reduced and local inflammation controlled. If pain and neurologic findings persist, surgical release of the ligament on the front of the wrist may be necessary.

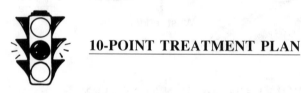 **10-POINT TREATMENT PLAN**

1. Activity Levels

- Moderate any wrist flexion activities such as typing and repetitive wrist activities.

2. Alternative Activities

- Routine sports activities such as running, biking, and swimming are generally not a problem.
- Excessive biking with the handlebar pressing on the wrist could cause a carpal tunnel.

3. Rehab Exercises

- Maintain wrist flexibility and work on strengthening exercises for the extensors of the wrist.
- See Upper Extremity Stretching Program, Beginning Tennis Elbow Program, and Advanced Tennis Elbow Program. Avoid any excessive bending that causes nerve symptoms.

4. Support

- Use a wrist cockup splint to keep the wrist in a neutral position, especially at sleeping time.

5. Thermal Treatment

- Use local ice massage to reduce pain and swelling about the wrist.

6. Medication

- Simple anti-inflammatory medicine such as aspirin or ibuprofen.
- Local steroid injection to reduce inflammation and swelling.

7. Equipment

- Use proper work and sports splints to avoid excessive flexion of the wrist.
- Sleep with simple wrist splint.

8. Nutrition

- Avoid obesity and follow a high-carbohydrate, low-fat diet.

9. Fluids

- Maintain hydration with proper fluid intake.

10. Surfaces

- This is generally not a problem in carpal tunnel syndrome, but avoid running on concrete to reduce jarring to the body.

14. Scaphoid Bone Fracture (Navicular Bone)

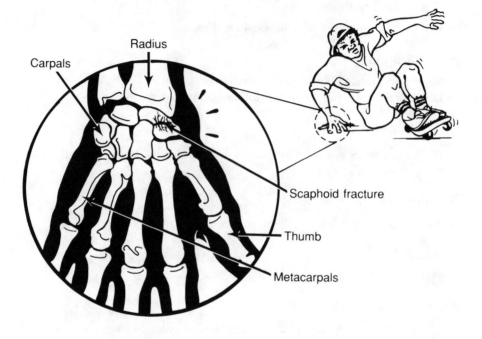

Radius

Carpals

Scaphoid fracture

Thumb

Metacarpals

6-POINT CONDITION SUMMARY

Definition

A traumatic condition on the thumb (radial) side from a fall on the hand, resulting in a fracture of the bone.

Cause

- An acute trauma to the wrist, generally from a fall (rarely a traumatic overuse) condition).

Subjective Symptoms

- Immediate and intense pain following a fall. Can be misinterpreted as a sprain.
- Swelling on the radial side of the wrist.
- Stiffness very pronounced.

Scaphoid Bone Fracture (Navicular Bone)

Objective Findings

- Tenderness is well localized on the thumb (radial) side of the wrist between the thumb and the wrist (the anatomical snuff box, the space between the thumb tendons).
- Stiffness and loss of motion exists.
- Nerve and vascular testing is normal.

Testing Procedures

- X-rays should be carefully examined for a fracture of the scaphoid.
- Initial X-ray may be normal.
- Bone scan in a few days will show a possible fracture at the bone.
- MRI may be helpful.
- Even if all tests are negative, but there is a strong clinical suspicion, the patient should be treated for a fractured scaphoid.

Prognosis

The most important part of the case is early diagnosis and immobilization. Cast immobilization in either a short-arm or long-arm cast is recommended. The blood flow to this bone is very poor at times, and eventual surgery with a bone graft may be indicated in a small percentage of cases. If not treated properly, degenerative arthritis of the wrist may form.

 10-POINT TREATMENT PLAN

1. Activity Levels

- Complete rest with splinting and casting of the wrist is required.
- General body activity is permitted.

2. Alternative Activities

- During the cast immobilization period, walking, swimming, and biking are allowed. A plastic bag on the cast may be used during swimming.

3. Rehab Exercises

- During cast immobilization, maintain isometric muscle tightening, exercises, and mobilization of the shoulder.

Scaphoid Bone Fracture (Navicular Bone)

- During cast immobilization, use Upper Extremity Stretching Program. Maintain general strength of the elbow and shoulder by using Advanced Tennis Elbow Program, but only with physician's approval because of the possibility of delayed union of the fracture.

4. Support

- During the first aid period, splinting is indicated, followed by a cast. Some surgeons recommend a short-arm cast, and some prefer a long-arm cast.

5. Thermal Treatment

- Use local ice initially for pain and swelling.
- Heat is not indicated because of the fracture and because it may cause more swelling.

6. Medication

- For the initial pain, codeine or narcotic injections are sometimes required.
- During cast immobilization, aspirin or anti-inflammatory medication may be indicated to reduce pain and swelling.
- Steroid injection is not indicated.

7. Equipment

- During the cast phase, biking may be used to maintain aerobic exercise.

8. Nutrition

- Maintain a high-carbohydrate, low-fat diet.

9. Fluids

- Maintain proper hydration with good fluid intake.

10. Surfaces

- Running on nonjarring surfaces is indicated during the cast immobilization period.

15. Ulnar Neuritis (Biker's Wrist)

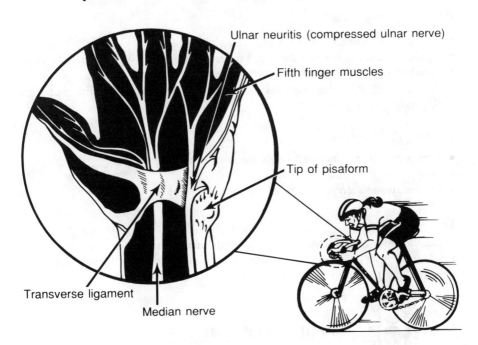

Ulnar neuritis (compressed ulnar nerve)

Fifth finger muscles

Tip of pisaform

Transverse ligament

Median nerve

6-POINT CONDITION SUMMARY

Definition

A local traumatic condition, usually in bikers, due to local pressure on the ulnar aspect (little finger side) of the wrist, resulting in pain and numbness in the fourth and fifth fingers.

Cause

- Acute violent trauma to the wrist in a fall or a direct hit on the ulnar aspect of the wrist.
- Chronic pressure in biking from leaning forward on the handlebar, with direct pressure on the ulnar aspect of the wrist.

Subjective Symptoms

- Pain in the wrist radiating to the fourth and fifth fingers.

- Numbness in the fourth and fifth fingers (ulnar nerve distribution) during biking.
- Weakness of the finger musculature.

Objective Findings

- Tenderness localized at the ulnar aspect of the wrist.
- Radiating numbness when the nerve is pressed or tapped—positive Tinel sign.
- Sensory loss in the fourth and fifth fingers.
- Weakness of the small muscles of the hand, especially the fourth and fifth fingers.

Testing Procedures

- X-rays are usually normal, but a small spur may be present.
- Bone scan is normal.
- MRI may show compression of the nerve.

Prognosis

Healing and reduction of pain occurs with change in pressure, padding of the wrist, and conservative measures. Some patients may require a local injection of steroid along the nerve. Surgery is possible but rarely done.

10-POINT TREATMENT PLAN

1. Activity Levels

- Reduce the amount of biking and pressure on the wrist.

2. Alternative Activities

- Running, swimming, and mountain biking are permissible.

3. Rehab Exercises

- Maintain muscle strength with hand grips.
- See Upper Extremity Stretching Program and, for wrist strengthening, Beginning Tennis Elbow Program and Advanced Tennis Elbow Program. Avoid any excessive stretching that causes nerve symptoms.

4. Support

- Padding of the bicycle handle and biking gloves.

5. Thermal Treatment

- Local ice after biking to reduce pain and numbness.

6. Medication

- Simple aspirin and ibuprofen for pain and inflammation.
- If pain persists, local injection of steroid.

7. Equipment

- Biking gloves that have special protection on the ulnar aspect of the wrist.
- Padded handlebars.
- Bicycle with an upright position such as a mountain bike.

8. Nutrition

- Maintain a high-carbohydrate, low-fat diet.

9. Fluids

- Maintain proper hydration with good fluid intake.

10. Surfaces

- Bicycle on smooth surfaces and avoid any bouncing and rough terrain.

16. Extensor Tendon Tear (Baseball Finger)

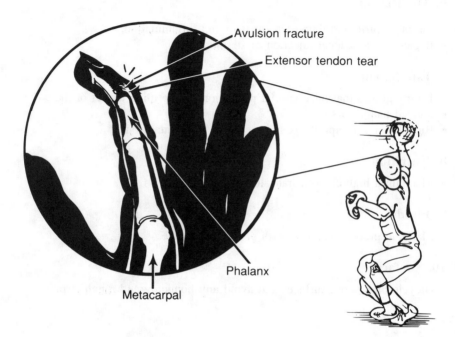

Avulsion fracture

Extensor tendon tear

Phalanx

Metacarpal

6-POINT CONDITION SUMMARY

Definition

A traumatic condition caused by direct, violent flexion to the tip of the finger, resulting in tear of the tendon (and possible bone fracture).

Cause

- Acute trauma when a ball (baseball) hits and suddenly flexes the tip of the finger, tearing the extensor (straightening) tendon and in some cases breaking off a piece of bone.
- Chronic repetitive bending in an elderly person leading to microtears in the tendon.

Subjective Symptoms

- Sudden pain at the tip of the finger (dorsal aspect).
- Swelling localized to the extensor side of the finger.

Extensor Tendon Tear (Baseball Finger)

- Inability to straighten the tip of the finger. Fingertip appears bent (mallet finger).

Objective Findings

- Tenderness localized to the dorsal tip of the finger.
- Local swelling present at the tip of the finger.
- Weakness in extension.
- Nerve exam normal.

Testing Procedures

- X-rays are normal if the tendon alone is torn. A bone injury may appear if a fracture is present.
- Bone scan and MRI are not needed.

Prognosis

Early treatment and diagnosis are vital to restoring tendon function. Splinting, casting, or pinning with open surgery may be chosen, depending on the extent of injury and the philosophy of the surgeon.

 10-POINT TREATMENT PLAN

1. Activity Levels

- The hand must be put to rest to avoid further displacement of the fracture.

2. Alternative Activities

- Running and biking are permitted to maintain aerobic fitness.

3. Rehab Exercises

- During periods of splinting, maintain upper-body strength and flexibility.
- See Upper Extremity Stretching Program and, for wrist strengthening, Beginning Tennis Elbow Program and Advanced Tennis Elbow Program. Exercises should be done very cautiously and only when prescribed by a physician because of the possibility of tearing the tendon.

4. Support

- Keep the finger splinted in extension either with a tongue blade or a plastic, commercially prepared extension splint. This is required for 4 to 8 weeks.

Extensor Tendon Tear (Baseball Finger)

5. Thermal Treatment

- Local ice to reduce pain and swelling.

6. Medication

- Codeine may be needed for the first 2 days, followed by simple aspirin or ibuprofen.

7. Equipment

- The finger should be splinted promptly in extension (straight).

8. Nutrition

- High-carbohydrate, low-fat diet.

9. Fluids

- Maintain good hydration.

10. Surfaces

- Activities should be done on a nonskid surface so the person does not fall on an outstretched hand.

17. Rupture Ulnar Collateral Ligament (Skier's Thumb)

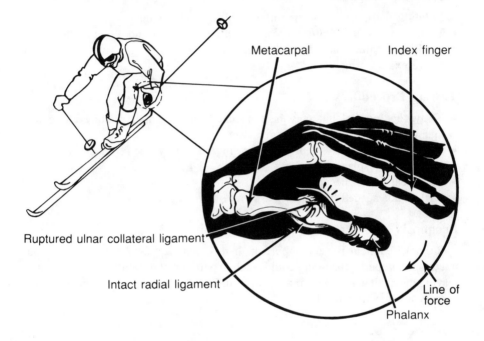

Metacarpal

Index finger

Ruptured ulnar collateral ligament

Intact radial ligament

Line of force

Phalanx

6-POINT CONDITION SUMMARY

Definition

A traumatic condition caused when the skier's outstretched hand falls onto a ski pole, resulting in a tear of the thumb ligament. Produces an unstable thumb and can lead to permanent disability.

Cause

- An acute tear of the ulnar ligament at the base of the thumb, generally during skiing, with the thumb bent outward from falling on the handle of the ski pole.
- Chronic stretching of the ligament from repeated minor stresses to the thumb (gamekeeper's thumb—caused by repeated snapping of the heads of small animals).

Subjective Symptoms

- Sudden pain at the base of the thumb during a fall.
- Inability to sustain a pinch between the thumb and the index finger.

Rupture Ulnar Collateral Ligament (Skier's Thumb)

- Local swelling at the base of the thumb.
- Nerve symptoms rare.

Objective Findings

- Instability at the base of the thumb with manual testing.
- Tenderness localized at the ulnar aspect (small finger side) of the thumb.
- Swelling localized at the ulnar aspect of the thumb.
- Nerve exam normal.

Testing Procedures

- X-rays are normal but may be associated with a small fracture along the ligament.
- Stress X-rays are very helpful for showing instability (the physician manually attempts to displace the joint).
- Bone scan is not needed.
- MRI is not needed but could show the ligament tear.

Prognosis

Prompt treatment is very important. If misdiagnosed as a simple sprain and not treated properly, the injury could result in permanent instability and disability, leaving the hand with a weak pinch and pain. Early splinting, casting, and possible surgery are recommended.

 10-POINT TREATMENT PLAN

1. Activity Levels

- Stop skiing at first and seek proper treatment and diagnosis.
- During casting, light aerobic activities such as light skiing can be maintained if proper protective splint has been applied.

2. Alternative Activities

- Other activities such as biking, swimming, and running can be performed.
- Upper-body weight lifting for flexibility and strength can be done.

3. Rehab Exercises

- During splinting and casting, maintain grip strength with isometric exercises for the hand.

Rupture Ulnar Collateral Ligament (Skier's Thumb)

- See Upper Extremity Stretching Program and, for wrist strengthening, see Beginning Tennis Elbow Program and Advanced Tennis Elbow Program. Obtain a rubber ball and do progressive strengthening and gripping exercises.

4. Support

- Initially, the thumb should be properly splinted and casted until the extent of instability and disability can be assessed.
- Use a protective thumb splint when returning to sports.

5. Thermal Treatment

- Use local ice to reduce pain and swelling.
- Heat, which may cause more swelling and make casting difficult, should not be used because of the severity of the injury.

6. Medication

- Simple analgesics with codeine may be necessary for the first few days, followed by aspirin and anti-inflammatory medication.

7. Equipment

- Avoid ski pole straps that wrap around the thumb.
- Use ski poles that have plastic grips that fit around the wrist and hand.

8. Nutrition

- Maintain a high-carbohydrate, low-fat diet during rehabilitation.

9. Fluids

- Maintain proper hydration with good fluid intake.

10. Surfaces

- When returning to skiing, avoid hard moguls and hard bouncing until adequate strength has been regained.

18. Tear of Adductor Muscles (Inner Thigh)

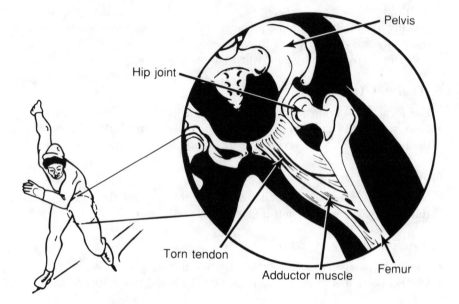

Pelvis

Hip joint

Torn tendon

Adductor muscle

Femur

6-POINT CONDITION SUMMARY

Definition

A traumatic muscle condition characterized by tearing or rupture of the adductor longus muscle (an inner muscle of the thigh that attaches to the pubic bone), resulting in local pain and limp.

Cause

- Sudden twisting and abduction (spreading the legs) in a high-impact twisting sport such as soccer or football.
- Tearing of the muscle group of the inner thigh.

Subjective Symptoms

- A sudden pain and pulling of the inner muscle of the thigh.
- Nerve symptoms such as numbness generally not present.
- A limp, possibly very pronounced, and progressive swelling.

Tear of Adductor Muscles (Inner Thigh)

Objective Findings

- Marked restriction of hip motion.
- Local swelling, bleeding, and hematoma (collection of blood).
- Neurologic exam usually normal.
- Muscle defects sometimes felt.

Testing Procedures

- Initial X-rays are usually normal.
- Nerve tests are usually normal.
- Specialized testing such as MRI is generally not indicated but may show a muscle defect.
- After several months, X-rays may show muscle calcification.

Prognosis

If tearing is in the muscle belly, healing may occur within weeks. If tearing is in the tendon where it attaches to the bone, healing may take months. Surgery rarely is necessary to repair the defect. Slow but progressive rehabilitation can be expected. Return to sports may take several months, depending on the extent of the tear.

 10-POINT TREATMENT PLAN

1. Activity Levels

- Straight activities are best, as dictated by the pain.
- Avoid twisting and sudden cutting maneuvers during the first several weeks of rehabilitation.
- Maintain muscle flexibility and strength.

2. Alternative Activities

- Walking, swimming, and biking are satisfactory when the pain is less intense.
- Run in a swimming pool with a Wet Vest for early rehabilitation.

3. Rehab Exercises

- Rest is the best initial treatment.
- If pain is mild, early walking, swimming, and biking are satisfactory.
- Isometric exercises with simple weights are helpful for maintaining muscle mass.

Tear of Adductor Muscles (Inner Thigh)

- As pain gradually subsides, more aggressive muscle rehabilitation in the form of isokinetic exercise machines may be used.
- See Lower Extremity Stretching Program and Lower Extremity Strengthening Program.

4. Support

- Wrapping the thigh, taping the thigh, or using a special elastic wrap in the upper thigh is helpful.
- Be careful with compression if bleeding and swelling are pronounced.

5. Thermal Treatment

- Because of the initial pain and swelling, local ice massage is the best treatment.
- Local heat after several days reduces muscle spasms.

6. Medication

- Take simple anti-inflammatory medication along with codeine if pain is very serious.
- After several weeks and if a local trigger point is present, then an injection of Xylocaine and steroid may be of help.

7. Equipment

- Good supportive shoes are necessary for early walking.
- Thigh wraps are helpful for maintaining muscle support and minimizing swelling.

8. Nutrition

- Because of bed rest, avoid obesity. A low-fat, high-carbohydrate diet is best.

9. Fluids

- Maintain proper hydration during periods of rest and training to maintain muscle function and urinary flow.

10. Surfaces

- Avoid impact and twisting activities early.
- Avoid hills and rough terrain.
- Stay on blacktop and bicycle paths for exercise.

19. Stress Fracture of the Neck of the Femur

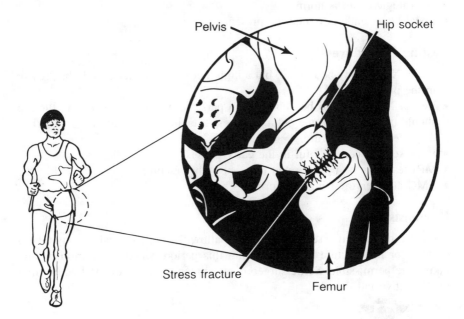

Pelvis

Hip socket

Stress fracture

Femur

6-POINT CONDITION SUMMARY

Definition

An overuse condition characterized by a localized weakening and cracking of the hip bone, due to repetitive lower extremity activities such as prolonged running on hard surfaces. Potentially a very serious problem that may require surgery if displacement of fracture is suspected or imminent.

Cause

- A prolonged running program on hard surfaces in a thin person, often a young woman, who is overtraining and losing weight.

Subjective Symptoms

- Progressive pain on the side, posterior aspect of the hip, or groin, with radiation into the inner thigh.
- Numbness and tingling usually not present.
- Muscle spasm present in some cases and confused with a simple muscle strain.
- Pain usually brought on by activities and relieved with rest and sitting.

Stress Fracture of the Neck of the Femur

Objective Findings

- Limp is present, especially with hopping and running.
- Motion is guarded on hip flexion and rotation.
- Neurologic exam is normal.
- Local bone tenderness may be present.

Testing Procedures

- Initial X-rays may be normal, but a high index of suspicion should be present in the physician.
- Repeat X-rays should be done if pain persists. All persistent pain in the hip should be X-rayed to rule out a hip stress fracture because of the serious risk: displacement of fracture.
- Bone scan is very helpful in the early phases.
- MRI test may be positive and may show the fracture.
- EMG and nerve testing are normal.

Prognosis

Generally good, if rest is prescribed to allow the bone to heal. It may take 3 months for the fracture to heal. During this period, walking, swimming, and biking are permissible. Some surgeons recommend pinning of the fracture in a highly active individual.

10-POINT TREATMENT PLAN

1. Activity Levels

- Avoid any impact or twisting activity. Err on the side of overresting.
- As pain subsides, gradually increase walking, swimming, and biking.

2. Alternative Activities

- Running in a swimming pool with a Wet Vest is allowed.
- Upper-body strengthening is allowed.
- Progress from walking, through race walking, to jogging.

3. Rehab Exercises

- Rest is especially indicated.
- Avoid any activity that causes pain.
- If walking, swimming, and biking are painless, they may be done with moderation.
- Maintain muscle strengthening with simple free weights.

Stress Fracture of the Neck of the Femur

- See Lower Extremity Stretching Program and Lower Extremity Strengthening Program.

4. Support

- The main support is emotional support from family, friends, and coaches. Athletes with this injury become frustrated and depressed very rapidly.
- Braces about the hip are not helpful.

5. Thermal Treatment

- Ice and heat are generally not helpful. Rest is the key.
- If muscle spasm is present, heat can be tried.

6. Medication

- Generally not helpful and may mask the fracture.
- Simple anti-inflammatory medications for muscle spasm.

7. Equipment

- Avoid any shoes that break down easily.
- Use stable shoes with excellent shock-absorbing qualities.
- Nonimpact exercise machines are permitted if there is no pain.

8. Nutrition

- Avoid overeating during periods of frustration and depression.
- In the high intensity athlete, a low-fat, high-carbohydrate diet is best, perhaps with supplemental calcium and vitamin D.
- Women who are not menstruating properly should consult with a gynecologist knowledgeable in sports for possible estrogen therapy.

9. Fluids

- Maintain good hydration during periods of rest and training to maintain muscle function and urinary flow.

10. Surfaces

- Avoid any hills or firm surfaces during rehabilitation.
- Stay on blacktop and bicycle paths.
- Avoid any surfaces that cause pain.

20. Trochanteric Bursitis

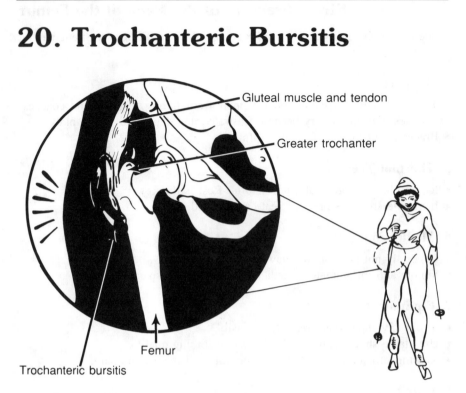

Gluteal muscle and tendon

Greater trochanter

Femur

Trochanteric bursitis

6-POINT CONDITION SUMMARY

Definition

Localized inflammation on the outer (lateral) side of the hip, characterized by local pain and limp, and common in aerobic sports.

Cause

- Long-distance running and biking cause the muscle-tendons to rub over the side of the hip bone, leading to irritation of the bursa.
- The athlete may have leg alignment problems (knock-knee), and shoes may have worn excessively on the lateral heel.

Subjective Symptoms

- Localized pain exists on the side of the hip.
- Local swelling may be present.
- Numbness and tingling are not present.
- Pain is relieved with rest.
- Sneezing and coughing are not painful.

Objective Findings

- Slight limp with running.
- Hip motion possibly guarded.
- Local tenderness directly on the side of the hip (trochanteric region).
- Neurologic exam normal.

Testing Procedures

- X-rays usually are normal but may show soft tissue calcifications.
- Specialized tests such as MRI, CAT scan, myelogram, and EMG are not necessary.
- Bone scan may be positive.

Prognosis

Healing generally occurs after initial rest. Symptoms may linger for several months. Surgery rarely is necessary; sometimes the bursa has to be excised and the tendon divided surgically, but this is unusual.

 10-POINT TREATMENT PLAN

1. Activity Levels

- Avoid extreme twisting during running.
- Maintain progressive straight aerobic activities such as moderate running and biking.

2. Alternative Activities

- Race walking, biking, and running in a swimming pool with a Wet Vest.

3. Rehab Exercises

- Extreme rest is not necessary. Let pain be the guide.
- Moderate running, biking, and swimming are very helpful.
- Avoid extreme long-distance running during periods of pain.
- Do simple weight lifting to strengthen the front and side muscles.
- Progressive isokinetic exercises are helpful with machines, but avoid torqueing the hip excessively.
- See Lower Extremity Stretching Program and Lower Extremity Strengthening Program.

4. Support

• Local wrap is generally not helpful.

5. Thermal Treatment

• Local ice massage is very helpful for reducing the swelling in the bursa.
• If muscle spasm is present, then heat may be used.

6. Medication

• Anti-inflammatory medication is helpful.
• Steroid injection is sometimes helpful for reducing the swelling in the bursa.

7. Equipment

• Avoid any lateral heel wear on the shoe. Wear firm-heeled shoes.

8. Nutrition

• Maintain a low-fat, high-carbohydrate diet.

9. Fluids

• Maintain good hydration during periods of rest and training to maintain muscle function and urinary flow.

10. Surfaces

• Avoid banks and hills and anything that will torque the hips.
• Stay on blacktop and bicycle paths for exercise.

21. Myositis Ossificans, Heterotopic Bone Formation

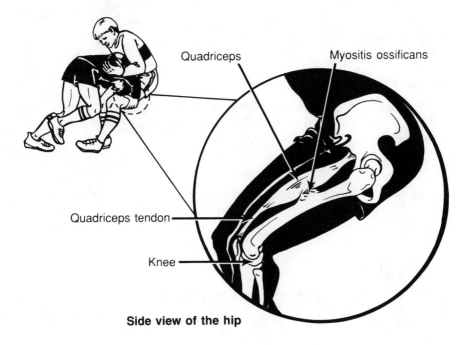

Quadriceps

Myositis ossificans

Quadriceps tendon

Knee

Side view of the hip

6-POINT CONDITION SUMMARY

Definition

A chronic soft-tissue inflammatory-traumatic condition with tearing and bleeding in the thigh muscle, resulting in abnormal scarring and extra bone formation ("myositis ossificans") directly inside the muscle. Generally starts as a simple muscle tear or bleed. If muscle not immobilized and rested, bone will form in it.

Cause

- A sudden impact or tearing of the quadriceps muscle.
- Lack of immobilization and rest in an injured muscle.

Subjective Symptoms

- Persistent pain several months after an injury to the thigh muscle.

Myositis Ossificans, Heterotopic Bone Formation

- Tightness and stiffness of the thigh muscle, with limitation of knee and hip motion.
- Stability excellent.
- A firm mass felt in some cases.

Objective Findings

- Well-localized tenderness and thickening of the muscle.
- Restriction in thigh and knee motion.
- A tender, swollen mass felt.

Testing Procedures

- X-rays show calcification and bone formation in the muscle.
- A bone scan and MRI may further document the problem.
- Arthroscopy is not helpful.

Prognosis

Aggressive physical therapy and many months of healing are required. Sometimes ultrasound helps to speed healing and reduce the inflammation. Surgery is rarely indicated. The long-term function is good, but healing period may be prolonged.

10-POINT TREATMENT PLAN

1. Activity Levels

- Let pain be the guide. Injury is caused by excessive activity during pain.

2. Alternative Activities

- Running, biking, swimming, and running in a swimming pool are all excellent ways of maintaining muscle function and aerobic activity.
- Forceful, heavy weight lifting is not indicated until the pain gradually subsides.

3. Rehab Exercises

- Straight-leg raising and bent-knee isometric exercises are indicated once the pain starts to subside.
- Do not force exercises and do not force stretching; this may cause more inflammation.

Myositis Ossificans, Heterotopic Bone Formation

- See Lower Extremity Stretching Program and Lower Extremity Strengthening Program. You must be very cautious with the exercise program because of the possibility of stimulating more bone growth. Careful monitoring by the physician and therapist are important.

4. Support

- Wrapping the thigh may help to maintain muscle compression and support.
- Wear a protective rubber pad on the thigh to prevent impact.

5. Thermal Treatment

- Ice during the acute muscle tear and bleed.
- In the chronic state, local heat to reduce muscle inflammation, along with a program of gentle exercise and rest.

6. Medication

- Simple anti-inflammatory medication is helpful.
- Local steroid injection may be helpful in the later phase of recovery.

7. Equipment

- Good shock-absorbing shoes.
- Isokinetic machines for gentle strength and flexibility.

8. Nutrition

- Avoid obesity. A high-carbohydrate, low-fat diet is very helpful.

9. Fluids

- Maintain a high fluid intake during exercise to prevent fatigue and muscle dehydration.

10. Surfaces

- Avoid running on hills or anything that excessively flexes the thigh.

22. Quadriceps Muscle Tear

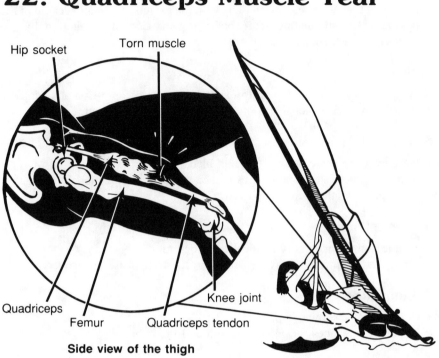

Hip socket — Torn muscle — Quadriceps — Femur — Knee joint — Quadriceps tendon

Side view of the thigh

6-POINT CONDITION SUMMARY

Definition

A traumatic muscle condition characterized by a sudden tearing of the muscle on the front of the thigh between the kneecap and hip joint, resulting in severe pain, limp, and inability to extend the knee.

Cause

- An acute contraction or sudden flexion of the thigh muscle, overloading the muscle strength and causing tear of the quadriceps muscle, often just above the kneecap.
- A chronic repetitive tearing due to excessive jumping or excessive overload with running or biking.

Subjective Symptoms

- Well-localized tenderness at the muscle-tendon junction, generally 2 or 3 inches above the kneecap.
- Local swelling in some cases.

- A sensation of giving way due to muscle weakness, especially if there is complete tear of the muscle.
- Jumping and kicking very painful.

Objective Findings

- Well-localized tenderness at the site of muscle tear.
- Limp present.
- Local swelling and bleeding.
- Weakness on extension of the knee.

Testing Procedures

- Routine X-rays are generally normal.
- MRI is generally not necessary but may show a tear of the muscle or tendon.
- Arthroscopy is not helpful.

Prognosis

Incomplete tears generally heal. If the diagnosis is not made initially and activity persists, calcification (called heterotopic bone formation or myositis ossificans) may form in the tendon. If there is a complete tear at the muscle-tendon junction, open surgical repair may be indicated.

 10-POINT TREATMENT PLAN

1. Activity Levels

- For a severe tear, surgery and rest are generally indicated.
- For incomplete tears, slow gradual walking, biking, and running are permissible. Avoid jumping and kicking.

2. Alternative Activities

- Early in recovery, swimming is permissible, especially if the leg is straight.
- Gradually progress to walking, biking, and light running.
- Hard jumping and kicking are the last activities.

3. Rehab Exercises

- Straight-leg-raising exercises and isometric contraction of the muscle are permissible early if no major tear exists.
- In a few weeks, as pain subsides, start gentle flexion exercises with isokinetic machines. Let pain be the guide.

- See Lower Extremity Stretching Program and Lower Extremity Strengthening Program. During the initial period of rehabilitation see the Patellar Program for strengthening exercises with the leg straight. Gradually progress to bent-knee exercises on the recommendation of your physician.

4. Support

- For incomplete tear, wrap the thigh with large elastic wraps.
- Rubber protective pad to the front of the thigh helps prevent impact injuries in basketball and football.

5. Thermal Treatment

- Local ice massage and compression.
- Heat in a few days as pain and swelling subside.

6. Medication

- Simple anti-inflammatory medication is indicated.
- After several months, a local steroid injection may be helpful at trigger points.

7. Equipment

- Generally, sports equipment is not a factor.
- Keep bicycle seat high.

8. Nutrition

- Avoid obesity. A low-fat, high-carbohydrate diet is very helpful.

9. Fluids

- Maintain fluid intake during exercise to prevent fatigue and muscle dehydration.

10. Surfaces

- Avoid running on hills and climbing stairs.
- Do activities on straight paths.

23. Hamstring Muscle Tear

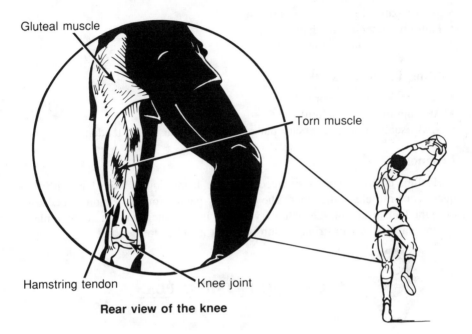

Gluteal muscle

Torn muscle

Hamstring tendon   Knee joint

Rear view of the knee

6-POINT CONDITION SUMMARY

Definition

A traumatic muscle condition characterized by a sudden tearing of the muscles of the posterior or hamstring. Tear usually located in the central portion of the thigh or the tendons at the knee or hip. Results in acute localized pain, limp, and inability to run.

Cause

- A sudden extension or violent jumping activity, overloading the muscle and causing an acute tear.
- A chronic, repetitive overuse condition due to tight muscle associated with running, biking, and jumping.

Subjective Symptoms

- Well-localized sharp pain in the muscle belly or pain near the knee or hip.
- Local swelling and bleeding present in some cases.
- Stability good, but pain with jumping.

Objective Findings

- Well-localized tenderness.
- Well-localized swelling and bruising.
- Pain on stretching the hamstring.
- Neurologic exam normal.

Testing Procedures

- Routine X-rays are normal.
- Arthrogram is not helpful.
- MRI usually is not necessary but may show a tear of the tendon.

Prognosis

Healing is often more prolonged with the hamstring tendon than with the quadriceps muscle in the front. The pain may persist for many months because of tight hamstring muscles. Surgery rarely is indicated, except for complete severe tear of the hamstring tendon where it attaches to the knee.

10-POINT TREATMENT PLAN

1. Activity Levels

- Early biking, swimming, and walking are satisfactory.
- As pain gradually subsides, intense running or biking are permissible.
- Jumping and rapid twisting are the last activities to be considered.

2. Alternative Activities

- Running in a swimming pool is an excellent way of maintaining aerobic activity and reducing strain on the hamstring tendon.
- Avoid violent kicking.

3. Rehab Exercises

- Rest is indicated at first.
- Do isometric exercises with the leg straight for early pain.
- As pain subsides, gradually return to flexion and stretching exercises with isokinetic machines.
- See Lower Extremity Stretching Program and Lower Extremity Strengthening Program. Emphasis should be on the hamstring muscle group for strengthening and stretching.

4. Support

• Wrap the thigh with elastic wraps, which will help reduce the pull on the inflamed muscle and tendon.

5. Thermal Treatment

• Ice massage to reduce pain and swelling.
• Local heat after several days to reduce muscle soreness.

6. Medication

• Simple anti-inflammatory medications such as aspirin or ibuprofen.
• If pain persists after several months, a local steroid injection may be of help in an inflamed area.

7. Equipment

• Keep the heel elevated with a very thick-heeled running shoe to reduce the hamstring pull.
• Use machines (biking, rowing) to maintain muscle flexibility and strength.

8. Nutrition

• Avoid obesity. A low-fat, high-carbohydrate diet is best.

9. Fluids

• Maintain good hydration during periods of training to maintain muscle function.

10. Surfaces

• Avoid hills and twisting activities.
• Run on soft surfaces such as blacktops or bicycle paths.

24. Anterior Cruciate Ligament Tear

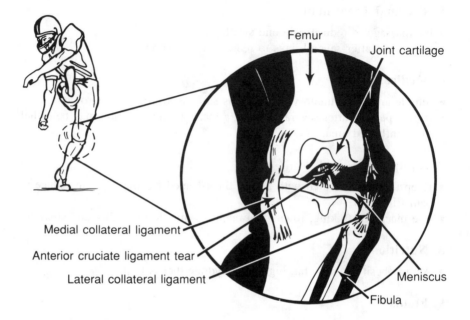

Femur

Joint cartilage

Medial collateral ligament

Anterior cruciate ligament tear

Lateral collateral ligament

Meniscus

Fibula

6-POINT CONDITION SUMMARY

Definition

A traumatic tearing of the main central ligament of the knee (anterior cruciate ligament), characterized by sudden twisting, giving way, and falling to the ground, causing a shifting and a "pop," with resulting disability. Can be serious condition requiring proper diagnosis, not just treated as a knee sprain.

Cause

- Acute twist and falling injury in jumping and twisting sports such as basketball, volleyball, and skiing.
- Chronic repeated microtrauma of many knee sprains leading to progressive tearing from incomplete to complete disruption.

Subjective Symptoms

- Pain either on the front or back of the knee.
- Swelling within 1 to 3 hours as blood accumulates.

Anterior Cruciate Ligament Tear

- A sensation of giving way and a shifting of the knee.
- Motion restricted as pain and swelling develop.
- Progressive limp and inability to jump.

Objective Findings

- Local tenderness on the front inner aspect of the knee.
- Swelling present due to blood in the knee.
- Instability tests such as Lachman, drawer, and pivot shift positive.
- Motion very restricted and limited in flexion and extension.

Testing Procedures

- Initial X-rays are normal but may show a small associated fracture. Chronic cases may show early signs of degenerative arthritis.
- MRI shows characteristic changes in the ligament and the meniscus.
- Arthrogram does not help to show the tear of the ligament but may show associated tears of the menisci.
- Arthroscopy is very diagnostic but should be reserved for severe cases.

Prognosis

Tears of the anterior cruciate ligament are an enigma. Healing of the torn ligament is unpredictable because of poor blood supply to the ligament. The prognosis depends on the extent of instability and the activity level of the athlete. There are many philosophies of treatment, ranging from muscle rehabilitation to sophisticated braces to complex open surgical procedures. Athletes should expect many months of rehabilitation before returning to twisting sports. This condition is a career-threatening injury, especially in basketball.

10-POINT TREATMENT PLAN

1. Activity Levels

- After the injury, rest is mandatory, but upper-body aerobic exercises are permissible.

2. Alternative Activities

- During rehabilitation, twisting sports should be avoided.
- Exercises that develop the thigh muscle should be done. The athlete may progress from walking, biking, and running in a swimming pool to jogging over a 3- to 6-month period.

3. Rehab Exercises

- For the acute tear, isometric exercises can be done to maintain muscle strength.
- During the rehabilitation phase, particular emphasis on the hamstring muscle is very important.
- For exercise, see Anterior Cruciate Knee Program.

4. Support

- Depending on the extent of instability, simple to very complex custom-made braces are advisable for stabilizing the knee.
- Braces are very effective in controlling the knee but are not a substitute for muscle rehabilitation and modification of activity.

5. Thermal Treatment

- Use ice for the first few days to reduce pain and swelling.
- Heat should not be used because it may aggravate the swelling of the knee. During rehabilitation, heat helps to maintain muscle relaxation.

6. Medication

- Codeine and Demerol may be necessary following the severe injury.
- This can be followed by aspirin and ibuprofen during the rehabilitation phase.

7. Equipment

- A good stabilizing shoe is very important for maintaining foot control during rehabilitation.
- Most exercise machines are satisfactory as long as they do not twist and torque the knee.

8. Nutrition

- Follow a high-carbohydrate, low-fat diet.

9. Fluids

- Maintain good hydration.

10. Surfaces

- Because of instability, curved rough surfaces should be avoided.
- Rough terrain must be avoided because it may lead to more instability.

25. Chondromalacia Patella

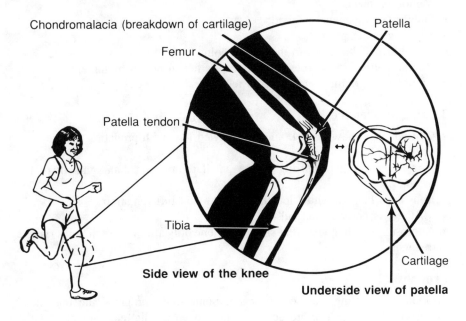

Chondromalacia (breakdown of cartilage)

Patella

Femur

Patella tendon

Tibia

Side view of the knee

Cartilage

Underside view of patella

6-POINT CONDITION SUMMARY

Definition

A traumatic or degenerative cartilage condition characterized by a local breakdown of the undersurface of cartilage, usually at the patella. Can be an early localized form of osteoarthritis or degenerative arthritis.

Cause

- Direct local trauma such as when the knee hits the dashboard in an automobile accident.
- Repeated bending microtrauma, especially if the joint is not aligned properly.

Subjective Symptoms

- Dull aching pain, leading to sharp localized pain in the front of the knee.
- Grinding sensation frequently.
- Swelling and fluid generally not present.
- Stiffness in squatting, bending, and climbing stairs.
- Sensation of giving way.

Objective Findings

- Motion is intact.
- Stability of ligaments is good.
- Swelling is not present.
- Tenderness is localized to the patella joint.
- Patella maltracking is present (kneecap is not in proper alignment).
- Crepitation (grinding sensation) is felt.

Testing Procedures

- Gait analysis shows knock knees or bowed legs with pronation (flat arches) of the feet.
- X-rays show slight spurring of the patellar joint and malalignment of the patella.
- Bone scan helps to show localized uptake and inflammation.
- MRI test is not very helpful.
- Arthroscopy is diagnostic but should be done only after failure of conservative treatment.

Prognosis

Good, but healing can be prolonged. Some cases progress and may need surgery in the form of arthroscopy or major open patella realignment.

10-POINT TREATMENT PLAN

1. Activity Levels

- Avoid bent-knee twisting activities such as aerobic dance or hard running up hills.
- Straight activities such as biking with high seat, walking, and slow running are best.

2. Alternative Activities

- Swimming and running in a swimming pool are excellent aerobic alternatives.
- Avoid the breaststroke (the frogkick).

3. Rehab Exercises

- Straight-leg-raising exercises with 5- to 10-pound weights are allowed.
- Avoid all excessive bent-knee activities.
- See Lower Extremity Stretching Program and Patellar Program.

4. Support

- Use a patella brace (an elastic sleeve with cutout for the patella).

5. Thermal Treatment

- Local ice massage best.
- Heat for muscle spasm.

6. Medication

- Take simple anti-inflammatory medications such as aspirin or ibuprofen.
- Local steroid injections are generally not helpful.

7. Equipment

- Wear firm-heeled antipronation shoes.
- Consider custom-made orthotics (arch supports) for shoes.

8. Nutrition

- Avoid obesity. A low-fat, high-carbohydrate diet is best.

9. Fluids

- Maintain good hydration during periods of training to maintain muscle function.

10. Surfaces

- Avoid hills and banked tracks.
- Use flat, soft surfaces like blacktop or bicycle paths for exercises.

26. Iliotibial Band Syndrome

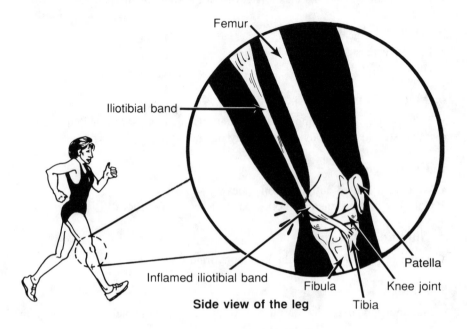

Femur

Iliotibial band

Inflamed iliotibial band

Side view of the leg

Patella

Fibula

Knee joint

Tibia

6-POINT CONDITION SUMMARY

Definition

An overuse inflammatory condition of the outer (lateral) aspect of the knee, characterized by an ache and burning sensation during or after running. Due to local friction of a tendon band as it rubs over the outer bone of the knee (lateral condyle).

Cause

- Acute, local, direct trauma. A rare cause.
- Chronic, overuse microtrauma, usually early in training in sports such as running or biking. Pain usually not disabling.

Subjective Symptoms

- Pain is well localized to the side of the knee on the outer flare of the bone. The pain may radiate up the side of the thigh to the hip.
- Swelling is not usually present.
- Motion is normal, but tightness may be perceived.
- Snapping may be present.

Objective Findings

- Tenderness is well localized to the band directly over the outer lateral condyle.
- Swelling is generally not present.
- Crepitation and noise are not usually present.
- Instability is not present.
- Knee exam is normal.
- Tightness of the lateral muscles may be present.

Testing Procedures

- X-rays are generally normal.
- Bone scan may be positive in chronic cases showing bone inflammation.
- MRI is not indicated.
- Arthroscopy is not indicated.

Prognosis

Progressive healing occurs with simple reduction in activity and muscle rehabilitation. The athlete may continue moderate biking and running during this condition. Surgery to split the tendon may be done in rare cases.

10-POINT TREATMENT PLAN

1. Activity Levels

- The athlete does not have to stop running but should simply reduce the intensity during periods of pain.

2. Alternative Activities

- Biking and running in a swimming pool are excellent alternatives for the runner.
- Avoid running on hills.

3. Rehab Exercises

- Maintain muscle flexibility, endurance, speed, and strength with particular emphasis on stretching the lateral muscles of the thigh and knee.
- See Lower Extremity Stretching Program and Lower Extremity Strengthening Program.

4. Support

- Simple elastic wrap or Neoprene wrap around the knee may be helpful.
- Avoid wraps that are too tight; they may lead to more friction.

5. Thermal Treatment

- Local ice massage directly after running.
- Heat massage to relax muscles before activities.

6. Medication

- Simple aspirin and ibuprofen help to reduce inflammation.
- In rare cases a local steroid injection may be used after months of treatment to reduce local inflammation.

7. Equipment

- Work more on upper-body aerobic exercise, and rest the knee.
- Shoes tend to wear on the lateral side of the heel. Wear shoes that have firm outer heels to stabilize the heel during heel strike.

8. Nutrition

- Follow a high-carbohydrate, low-fat diet.

9. Fluids

- Maintain good hydration.

10. Surfaces

- Avoid running on hard, rough surfaces.

27. Osgood Schlatter's Disease

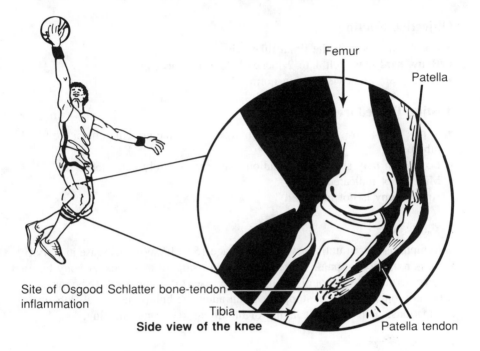

Femur

Patella

Site of Osgood Schlatter bone-tendon inflammation

Tibia

Side view of the knee

Patella tendon

6-POINT CONDITION SUMMARY

Definition

A traumatic tendon condition in a growing, active adolescent age 12 to 14. Condition characterized by pain where the tendon attaches to the shin bone (tibial tuberosity, a growth zone). Not really a disease.

Cause

- A sudden jump causing local tearing of the growth zone where the tendon attaches.
- Chronic: repetitive jumping, running, and bending in a young, growing adolescent. Just as in "jumper's knee," may be aggravated by leg and foot imbalance or excessive hill running.

Subjective Symptoms

- Pain: a progressive ache below the knee in activities such as jumping and hard running, usually in basketball.
- Swelling: a firm bump below the knee.

- Motion intact.
- Nerve symptoms not present.

Objective Findings

- Local tenderness at the tibial tuberosity.
- Bony, hard mass felt 1 to 2 inches below the kneecap.
- Knee exam otherwise within normal limits.

Testing Procedures

- X-rays show a fragmentation and enlargement of the growth zone at the tibial tuberosity.
- Bone scan may show inflammation, but scan is rarely indicated.
- MRI is not indicated.
- Arthroscopy is not indicated.

Prognosis

Symptoms persist until growth stops at age 16 or 17. With decrease in activity there is reduction in pain. There is no need to stop all activities. A bony bump may be permanent but not disabling. In rare cases the bump needs to be removed surgically once growth is stopped. As an adult the bump may be a problem in occupations, such as carpet laying or plumbing, requiring kneeling.

10-POINT TREATMENT PLAN

1. Activity Levels

- Moderate reduction in activity is needed, but there is no need to stop activities. This is not a disease and is not a serious condition.

2. Alternative Activities

- Try to avoid hard jumping sports.
- Moderate biking, swimming, and running are permitted.

3. Rehab Exercises

- Maintain flexibility, endurance, speed, and strength with moderate biking and weight lifting.
- Do the general stretching exercises in the Lower Extremity Stretching Program. Add the Patellar Program.

Osgood Schlatter's Disease

4. Support

- Simple elastic wrap or Neoprene sleeve around the knee will help reduce the pressure on the bone center.

5. Thermal Treatment

- Local ice massage after sports activities.
- Heat before sports to relax muscles.

6. Medication

- Pills generally are not necessary, but simple aspirin or Tylenol can be taken.

7. Equipment

- Use good stabilizing shoes to prevent foot imbalance.

8. Nutrition

- A high-carbohydrate, low-fat diet is recommended.

9. Fluids

- Maintain good hydration.

10. Surfaces

- Play basketball and run on soft surfaces.
- Avoid concrete for sports.
- Avoid running on curved surfaces.

28. Osteoarthritis

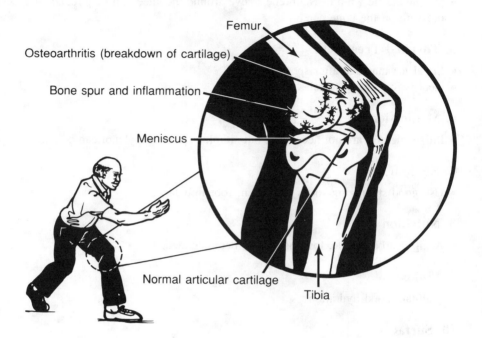

Femur

Osteoarthritis (breakdown of cartilage)

Bone spur and inflammation

Meniscus

Normal articular cartilage

Tibia

6-POINT CONDITION SUMMARY

Definition

A traumatic or degenerative condition of the cartilage of the knee joint, characterized by progressive wearing of the articular surface (hyaline cartilage). Progressive pain and stiffness. Bone spur formation gives the condition the name osteoarthritis. Progressive deterioration because of poor circulation to cartilage.

Cause

- Acute: traumatic injury to the surface of the joint from an impact or a twisting injury.
- Chronic: years of microtrauma to a joint, especially if malalignment or instability is present, such as with a torn anterior cruciate ligament.
- Other causes: obesity, idiopathic (cause not known) changes, and hereditary factors.

Subjective Symptoms

- Pain and ache are present after activity. The pain may be delayed until the next day or night.

- Swelling may be present in or around the joint.
- A sensation of giving way may be present while climbing stairs.
- Crepitation and noise can be felt and heard by the patient.
- Limp progressively develops.

Objective Findings

- Tenderness is present directly on the joint and along bone spurs.
- Swelling and fluid accumulation can be perceived.
- Crepitation can be felt and heard by the physician.
- Stiffness and loss of motion are detected.
- Limp is present with weight bearing and jumping.

Testing Procedures

- Initial X-rays are normal, even though cartilage is wearing. As the condition worsens, X-rays reveal roughness, narrowing of joint line, and spur formation.
- Bone scan is very helpful for detecting bone inflammation.
- MRI may show tears of the meniscus and wearing of the cartilage.
- Arthroscopy will definitely show defects in the hyaline cartilage, but generally the test is not used early to establish the diagnosis. Arthroscopy may be helpful in treating moderate cases by smoothing roughened surfaces and removing loose bodies.

Prognosis

Progressive deterioration of the joint will occur if you do not listen to your body. Pain indicates that progressive wearing is occurring. Reduce the intensity of activities until pain is minimal. Moderation of activity and intensity is very important. Twisting sports should be minimized. Nonimpact activities such as biking, walking, and swimming are satisfactory. Surgery, ranging from arthroscopy to eventual total joint replacement, may be required if the condition is very serious.

10-POINT TREATMENT PLAN

1. Activity Levels

- Nonimpact activities are the best.
- Avoid any exercise that causes discomfort directly in the joint.

2. Alternative Activities

- Swimming, biking, and walking are the best.

3. Rehab Exercises

- Maintain muscle strength and flexibility with moderate, nonimpact exercises.
- Gentle weight lifting, swimming, and biking are permissible.
- See Lower Extremity Stretching Program and Lower Extremity Strengthening Program. For range of motion add the Meniscus Knee Program.

4. Support

- The best support is muscle development.
- During periods of pain and swelling, a simple elastic wrap or brace can be used around the inflamed joint.
- Cane—for limp.

5. Thermal Treatment

- During period of acute pain and swelling, ice is preferred.
- Use heat for local muscle tightness and stiffness of the joint.

6. Medication

- Aspirin and ibuprofen should be the first line of defense.
- Nonsteroidal anti-inflammatory medications may be prescribed by your physician.
- Local steroid injection and aspiration may be intermittently tried but should be kept to a minimum.

7. Equipment

- Use stable, firm-heeled shoes.
- Avoid equipment that excessively bends the joint.

8. Nutrition

- It is very important to avoid obesity and progressive loss in muscle.
- A high-carbohydrate, low-fat diet is important. It is also important to maintain protein levels if you are middle-aged or elderly.

9. Fluids

- Maintain good hydration.

10. Surfaces

- It is very important to avoid hard, rough surfaces during walking, running, and sporting activities.

29. Kneecap (Patella) Dislocation

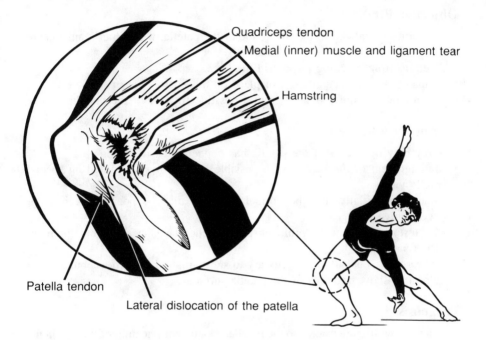

Quadriceps tendon

Medial (inner) muscle and ligament tear

Hamstring

Patella tendon

Lateral dislocation of the patella

6-POINT CONDITION SUMMARY

Definition

A traumatic condition in which the kneecap (patella) slides or shifts to the outer (lateral) side of the knee, either momentarily (until the patella replaces itself) or for a prolonged period (until a physician reduces it).

Cause

- Acute: a fall or direct trauma to the front and inner side of the kneecap, resulting in tearing of the inner ligaments, which stabilize the patella.
- Chronic: usually in an adolescent female with malalignment (knock knees) and lax ligaments, resulting in a shift of the patella in a twisting sport.

Subjective Symptoms

- Pain localized to the front and inner side of the patella.
- Swelling of the knee present due to bleeding.

- Kneecap perceived to be out of place in some cases.
- A sensation of giving way as the patella slides out of place.
- Grinding sensation present because of injury to the surface of the patella.

Objective Findings

- Tenderness localized to the inner side of the patella, where the ligaments are torn.
- Swelling from bleeding present in the knee.
- A mass perceived. Patella out of place on the lateral side of the knee.
- Crepitation and noise present from a possible fracture of the patella.

Testing Procedures

- X-ray may be normal if the patella has popped back in place.
- Malalignment of the patella with possible fracture may be noted on special patella views.
- Bone scan initially may be normal but later may be positive because of degenerative changes.
- MRI test is usually not helpful, but special techniques may show malalignment of the patella.
- Arthroscopy is usually not necessary to substantiate the diagnosis but may be helpful to show fractures of the patella surface.

Prognosis

In a male with acute trauma to the patella, spontaneous healing of the ligaments and muscles usually occurs without recurrence of the dislocation. In a female with laxity and malalignment, recurrent dislocation may occur, requiring limitation in sports and possible surgery to realign the patella.

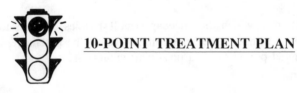

10-POINT TREATMENT PLAN

1. Activity Levels

- Rest the knee and avoid any flexion activities during the acute healing phase.

2. Alternative Activities

- Upper-body exercises such as with the Aerodyne bicycle are permitted. Biking with the good leg is permitted. Place the painful knee on a chair or on a bicycle bar.

3. Rehab Exercises

- Avoid any activities that flex the knee and stress the patella.
- Maintain muscle and quadriceps strength with straight-leg-raising exercises, and use a patellar rehabilitation program.
- See Lower Extremity Stretching Program and Lower Extremity Strengthening Program. See also Patellar Program.

4. Support

- The knee should be immobilized in extension (straight) for 2 to 4 weeks in either a cast or a knee immobilizer.
- During the rehabilitation phase, special patella harnesses and braces help to maintain the proper position of the patella until muscle rehabilitation is complete.

5. Thermal Treatment

- Use ice initially to reduce pain and swelling.
- During the rehabilitation phase, heat may be used for muscle relaxation.

6. Medication

- During acute injury, 1 or 2 days of codeine may be required, followed by aspirin or ibuprofen.
- The knee may need to be aspirated of the blood and possibly injected with an anti-inflammatory medication because of recurrent fluid formation.

7. Equipment

- During the initial healing phase, avoid any exercise that flexes the knees—for example, biking, running, or heavy weight lifting.

8. Nutrition

- Avoid obesity during the immobilization period.
- A high-carbohydrate, low-fat diet is recommended.

9. Fluids

- Maintain good hydration.

10. Surfaces

- During rehabilitation, do light sports on nonskid surfaces.
- Biking and running should be on smooth, soft surfaces that will not jar or twist the knee.

30. Patellar Tendinitis (Jumper's Knee)

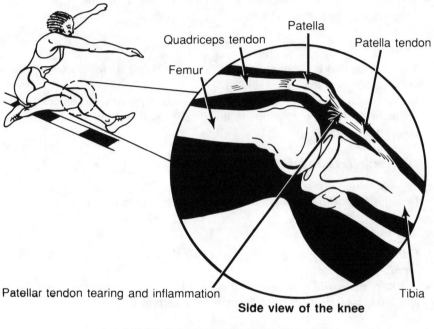

Quadriceps tendon

Patella

Patella tendon

Femur

Patellar tendon tearing and inflammation

Tibia

Side view of the knee

6-POINT CONDITION SUMMARY

Definition

A traumatic inflammation of the tendon directly below the kneecap (patella), initiated by jumping or climbing sports and resulting in incomplete local tearing of the tendon. Prolonged symptoms common for many months because of poor blood supply and resulting inflammation.

Cause

- Acute, violent jumping episode results in pain below the kneecap (patella) and leads to chronic pain and inflammation.
- Chronic, repetitive jumping, climbing, and running activities can weaken the tendon. Foot imbalance or running up hills are aggravating factors. "Slam dunking" is a frequent cause in basketball, especially in the leg responsible for push-off during the jump.

Patellar Tendinitis (Jumper's Knee)

Subjective Symptoms

- Pain localized to the tip of the bone just below the kneecap.
- Swelling generally not present.
- Motion within normal limits.
- Noise and crepitation generally not present.
- Giving way present with hard jumping.

Objective Findings

- Tenderness directly on the lower tip of the kneecap.
- Swelling generally not present.
- Crepitation not present.
- Instability not present.

Testing Procedures

- X-rays are normal, but a spur may be present in chronic cases.
- Bone scan may be positive at the inferior (lower) pole of the patella.
- In chronic cases, MRI may show an incomplete tear and a chronic tendon problem.
- Arthroscopy is not indicated.

Prognosis

Expect many months to a year in some cases for complete healing. Some cases never heal in basketball players. Chronic restriction in jumping may be present for 1 or 2 years. Some patients require surgery to remove scarred tendon. This can affect the long-term playing ability of a volleyball or basketball athlete.

10-POINT TREATMENT PLAN

1. Activity Levels

- Since this is *jumper's knee*, restrict jumping and hard running.

2. Alternative Activities

- Swimming and biking help to maintain aerobic conditioning.

3. Rehab Exercises

- Maintain flexibility, endurance, speed, and strength with a patella exercise program.

Patellar Tendinitis (Jumper's Knee)

- Do Lower Extremity Stretching Program and Lower Extremity Strengthening Program. See also Patellar Program.

4. Support

- Neoprene or elastic sports bandages around the patella help reduce the forces on the tendon.
- Orthotics (arch supports) for the shoes help to maintain foot control.

5. Thermal Treatment

- Ice after activities to reduce inflammation.
- Heat before sports to maintain muscle flexibility.

6. Medication

- Aspirin, ibuprofen, and other nonsteroidal anti-inflammatory medications are helpful, but be cautious because of the chronic nature of this problem.
- A local steroid injection may be helpful, but the tendon should not be injected directly. Frequent injections may further weaken and tear the tendon.

7. Equipment

- Avoid machines such as bikes or rowing machines that excessively bend the knee.
- Use shoes with excellent pronation control.
- An orthotic (arch support) may be necessary for the shoe if foot imbalance is present.

8. Nutrition

- Maintain a high-carbohydrate, low-fat diet.

9. Fluids

- Maintain good hydration.

10. Surfaces

- Avoid hills or rough surfaces, which torque and stress the patella.

31. Torn Meniscus

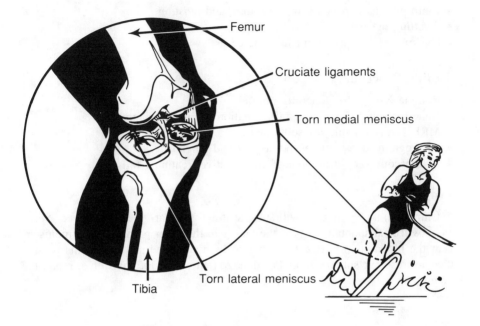

Femur

Cruciate ligaments

Torn medial meniscus

Torn lateral meniscus

Tibia

6-POINT CONDITION SUMMARY

Definition

A traumatic cartilage condition associated with wearing and eventual tearing of the fibrocartilage (the meniscus), the main shock absorber of the knee and the structure that provides cushioning between the femur and the tibia.

Cause

- Acute twisting trauma such as a hard flexion or rotation injury in basketball or soccer.
- A chronic overuse condition from repetitive bending and frequent twisting.

Subjective Symptoms

- Well-localized tenderness on the joint line, leading to progressive pain and swelling.
- Locking of the joint a feature in some cases.
- Stability good, but a sensation of giving way present in some cases.

Objective Findings

- Tenderness well localized at the joint line.
- Limp present, especially with bending and twisting.
- Swelling present.
- Clicking sensation present in some cases.

Testing Procedures

- Routine X-rays are generally normal.
- Bone scan will show local inflammation but is not diagnostic.
- MRI is very reliable for subtle tear.
- Arthrogram (dye test) can be helpful and diagnostic.
- Arthroscopy should be done if conservative treatment fails.

Prognosis

Untreated, the symptoms will subside if activities are greatly reduced. Some cases will heal spontaneously if the tear is in the outer portion of the meniscus near the blood supply. If activity has to be maintained and symptoms persist, then arthroscopic surgery should be done to remove the torn portion or repair the meniscus.

10-POINT TREATMENT PLAN

1. Activity Levels

- Let pain be the guide, and avoid any repeated, hard twisting bending maneuvers.

2. Alternative Activities

- Avoid ball sports, most of which require twisting.
- Walking, swimming, biking, and light running are satisfactory if pain is minimal.

3. Rehab Exercises

- Quadriceps and hamstring strengthening should be done with gentle weight lifting, using free weights or isokinetic machines.
- Let pain be the guide, and do not force exercise.
- See Lower Extremity Stretching Program and Meniscus Knee Program.

4. Support

- Bracing can help until muscle development is improved.
- Simple front-lace upbrace with simple metal hinges can help.

5. Thermal Treatment

- Local ice massage helps to relieve symptoms but generally will not correct the mechanical problem.

6. Medication

- Simple anti-inflammatory medication such as aspirin and ibuprofen is helpful.
- Local steroid injection sometimes helps to reduce the local synovitis and inflammation.

7. Equipment

- Avoid excessive lateral heel wear in the shoe.
- Use good, firm-heeled shoes.

8. Nutrition

- Avoid obesity. A high-carbohydrate, low-fat diet is very helpful.

9. Fluids

- Maintain fluid with high fluid intake during exercise to prevent fatigue and muscle dehydration.

10. Surfaces

- Avoid any rough surfaces that may twist the knee.
- Do most activities on straight paths.

32. Shin Splints

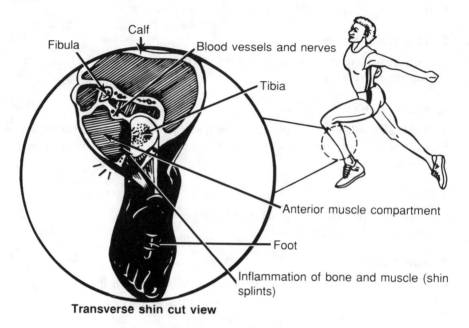

Transverse shin cut view

6-POINT CONDITION SUMMARY

Definition

An inflammation along the periosteum (outer lining of the bone), characterized by a diffuse pain along the front of the shin and due to repetitive stress.

Cause

- Associated with a foot imbalance and repetitive running on hard surfaces.
- If prolonged, may progress to a stress fracture.

Subjective Symptoms

- Diffuse pain along the inner side of the shin starts 2 or 3 inches below the knee and runs to the ankle.
- Thickening of the muscle belly and muscle tenderness can develop.
- Local swelling may be present.
- If swelling increases, nerve symptoms such as numbness and weakness of the foot can develop. This is known as *compartment syndrome*.

Objective Findings

- Diffuse and localized tenderness of the muscle and bone.
- Firmness of the muscle.
- Running with external rotation and a pronated foot.
- Late nerve damage detected in compartment syndrome in some cases.

Testing Procedures

- Routine X-rays are generally normal.
- Compartment testing, involving placement of a needle in the muscle, may show increased muscle pressure.
- MRI is not helpful.
- Bone scan may show diffuse bone inflammation and may help rule out a fracture.

Prognosis

Healing usually progresses as you reduce training, correct muscle imbalance, and treat inflammation. If healing is prolonged, a stress fracture can develop.

 10-POINT TREATMENT PLAN

1. Activity Levels

- Reduce running or jumping on hard surfaces.

2. Alternative Activities

- Running in a swimming pool is an excellent aerobic alternative.
- Biking, race walking, and cross-country skiing are excellent alternatives during the pain.

3. Rehab Exercises

- Rest if very painful, and reduce intensity of aerobic exercise.
- Gradually increase muscle strength and muscle flexibility with weights and rubber tubing.
- Progress to biking and swimming.
- See Ankle Program.

4. Support

- Wrap the shins with elastic wraps, or apply taping.
- Neoprene shin guards may be helpful.
- Be careful not to apply too much pressure; too much pressure may lead to a compartment syndrome.
- Wear a shoe with good arch support.

5. Thermal Treatment

- Ice massage to reduce pain and swelling after activity.
- Local heat before activity to relax muscles.

6. Medication

- Take simple anti-inflammatory medication such as aspirin or ibuprofen.
- If a local area of pain persists after several months, a local steroid injection may be given.

7. Equipment

- A stabilizing, shock-absorbing shoe.
- An arch support or an orthotic added to the shoe for foot imbalance.

8. Nutrition

- Avoid obesity. A low-fat, high-carbohydrate diet is best.

9. Fluids

- Maintain good hydration during periods of training to maintain muscle function.

10. Surfaces

- Avoid hills and rough terrain.
- Run on soft surfaces such as blacktop or bicycle paths.

33. Tibia or Fibula Stress Fracture

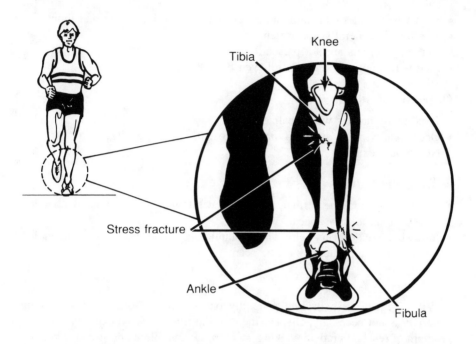

6-POINT CONDITION SUMMARY

Definition

A traumatic bone condition characterized by early persistent inflammation from shin splints, leading to persistent weakening of the bone and actual crack or fracture.

Cause

- Repetitive overuse associated with muscle imbalance and poor alignment of the leg, leading to actual weakening and fracture of the bone.
- Leg malalignment with foot pronation.
- Running on concrete roads with poor shoes.
- Eating disorder with excess weight loss.

Tibia or Fibula Stress Fracture

Subjective Symptoms

- Initial diffuse pain progresses to a well-localized point of pain, generally on the tibia on the inside of the shin or the outer aspect of the leg above the ankle (fibula bone).
- Vague pain and slight limp can progress to severe local pain and limp.
- Swelling is generally not present until late.
- Nerve symptoms are not present.
- Pain with impact and use is relieved by rest.

Objective Findings

- Bone tenderness is well localized.
- Occasionally, local swelling may be present.
- Neurologic exam is normal.

Testing Procedures

- Initial X-rays may be normal, but after several weeks a fracture and a healing bone formation may appear.
- Initial bone scan is very helpful in substantiating the diagnosis and in indicating prognosis by the intensity of the scan.

Prognosis

With adequate rest, healing generally occurs after 2 to 3 months. Casting generally is not necessary. Displacement of the fracture is very unusual. With a program of rest and gradual walking, swimming, and biking, progressive healing occurs. Long-term correction with foot correction device such as an orthotic is generally very helpful.

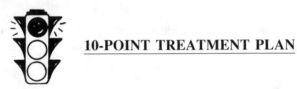

10-POINT TREATMENT PLAN

1. Activity Levels

- Initially, running must be curtailed.
- Avoid any activity that causes a limp or pain.

2. Alternative Activities

- Running in a swimming pool is an excellent way of maintaining aerobic activity and reducing impact on the bone.
- Race walking, cross-country skiing, and rowing are all permissible if very little pain is produced.

3. Rehab Exercises

- Inactivity and eliminating impact are key.
- Alternative walking and biking are permissible if pain is minimal.
- See Ankle Program and Lower Extremity Strengthening Program.

4. Support

- Wrapping an elastic bandage or Neoprene on the shin may help during early rehabilitation.

5. Thermal Treatment

- Ice massage initially, but this should not be a substitute for rest.

6. Medication

- Take simple anti-inflammatory medication such as aspirin or ibuprofen.
- Steroid injection is not indicated.
- Overmedication may mask the fracture.
- Calcium pills and vitamins not needed unless there is an eating disorder.
- Hormone therapy may be helpful if not menstruating properly.

7. Equipment

- A good, stable, antipronation shoe is very important for prevention.
- An orthotic arch support may be necessary to prevent foot imbalance.

8. Nutrition

- Avoid obesity, especially during the frustration of prolonged inactivity while the fracture is healing.
- Watch for and get help for any "eating disorder."
- A low-fat, high-carbohydrate diet is best.

9. Fluids

- Maintain good hydration during periods of training.

10. Surfaces

- Avoid concrete or hard paths during a running program.
- Avoid hills during the initial healing phase.

34. Rupture of the Gastrocnemius Muscle

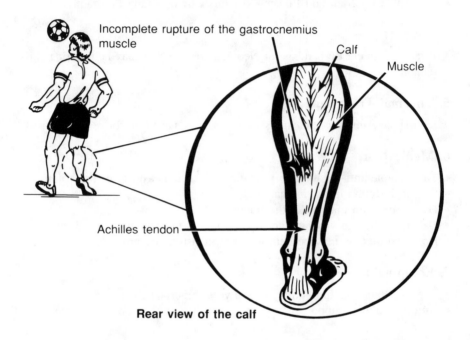

Incomplete rupture of the gastrocnemius muscle

Calf

Muscle

Achilles tendon

Rear view of the calf

6-POINT CONDITION SUMMARY

Definition

A traumatic muscle condition, typically in a middle-aged athlete and characterized by sudden partial tearing of the inner muscle belly of the calf, generally during a sudden jump as in tennis or basketball.

Cause

- Sudden violent jumping or pushing off, causing overloading and tearing of the muscle on the medial (inner) aspect of the muscle belly of the calf.
- Muscle tightness present, generally in a middle-aged male.

Subjective Symptoms

- Sudden onset of intense pain, as if you have been kicked or hit by a ball.
- Progressive limping and swelling.
- Symptoms reduced by using a heel lift.

Rupture of the Gastrocnemius Muscle

Objective Findings

- Well-localized pain, swelling, and hematoma (collection of blood).
- Nerve exam generally normal.
- Great difficulty walking on tiptoe.
- Achilles tendon mechanism intact (checked by squeezing the calf to see if it produces flexion of the foot).

Testing Procedures

- Initial X-rays are normal.
- MRI is generally not necessary but could possibly show a small tear of the muscle.
- Bone scan is negative.

Prognosis

Generally 6 to 8 weeks of healing are required. Once healed, the muscle tends to be normal, and recurrences are highly unusual. The main possible complication could be thrombophlebitis or blood clot formation, due to swelling and compression of veins. The condition tends to occur in middle-aged people who are developing increasing tightness and weakness. These two factors should be prevented.

 10-POINT TREATMENT PLAN

1. Activity Levels

- Early biking, swimming, and walking are satisfactory.
- Lift 5- to 10-pound ankle weights, increasing the weight gradually, to rehabilitate and maintain muscle strength, flexibility, and endurance.

2. Alternative Activities

- Running in a swimming pool is an excellent way of maintaining aerobic activity.
- Gentle biking with toe clips balances the force on the front and back of the thigh.

3. Rehab Exercises

- Rest is indicated during the first several weeks.
- Gentle biking, swimming, and walking can be done, especially with a heel lift.
- See Lower Extremity Strengthening Program and Ankle Program.

4. Support

- Add a heel lift.
- Wrap your ankle up to the calf with a light elastic bandage, but not too tight: Too tight a wrap may bring on phlebitis.

5. Thermal Treatment

- Local ice massage will reduce pain and swelling.
- If muscle spasm is severe, local heat can be used.

6. Medication

- Take simple anti-inflammatory medication such as aspirin or ibuprofen.
- If after several months a local area of pain persists due to tendinitis, a local steroid injection could be done.

7. Equipment

- Add a 1-inch heel lift to your shoe.
- A cane or crutch may be necessary.

8. Nutrition

- Avoid obesity. A low-fat, high-carbohydrate diet is best.

9. Fluids

- Maintain good hydration during periods of training to maintain muscle function.

10. Surfaces

- Avoid running up hills.
- Stay on soft surfaces such as blacktop or bicycle paths.

35. Achilles Tendinitis

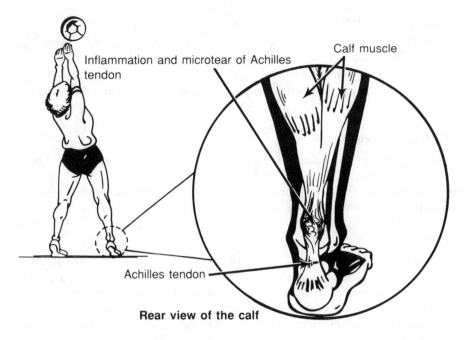

Inflammation and microtear of Achilles tendon

Calf muscle

Achilles tendon

Rear view of the calf

6-POINT CONDITION SUMMARY

Definition

A traumatic or degenerative tendon condition characterized by chronic pain and inflammation on the back of the ankle along the Achilles tendon, at the junction where the large muscle group of the calf attaches to the heel bone. Not a complete tear, but a partial tendon fiber disruption and inflammation.

Cause

- Acute, sudden jumping or running, causing a microscopic tearing of the muscle group, possibly in a previously weakened tendon.
- Chronic repetitive microtrauma to Achilles tendon, usually associated with muscle imbalance, excessive running up hills, or both. Foot imbalance present in some cases.

Subjective Symptoms

- Localized pain appears behind the ankle along Achilles tendon.
- Local thickening and swelling of the tendon may be present.

- Stiffness: The ankle may be tight, and pain may be aggravated by walking on the toes.

Objective Findings

- Well-localized tenderness appears directly on the Achilles tendon, either in the midsubstance of the tendon or where it attaches to the bone.
- Local swelling may be present.
- Muscle testing will induce pain on plantar flexion of the ankle and on walking on the toes.

Testing Procedures

- Routine X-rays are generally negative, but a small spur on the back of the heel may be present.
- Bone scan is not helpful but may show slight bone inflammation.
- MRI test may show tearing of the tendon in acute and chronic stages.

Prognosis

Healing can be prolonged because of poor circulation in the tendon. On a conservative program, slow but progressive healing may occur with incomplete or micro-chronic tears. If pain persists, open surgical removal of scar tissue in the tendon may be necessary. For acute tears, either casting or surgical treatment is indicated, depending on the activity level of the athlete and the philosophy of the surgeon.

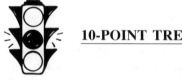 **10-POINT TREATMENT PLAN**

1. Activity Levels

- Proceed with caution. Let pain be the guide.
- Slow, gentle, light running is permissible, and try to avoid excessive jumping or propulsion exercises.

2. Alternative Activities

- Avoid hard jumping and twisting.
- Choose slow, gentle, straight activities such as race walking.
- Biking and swimming are satisfactory.

3. Rehab Exercises

- Do strengthening exercises for the front muscles of the shin and gentle stretching exercises for the calf muscle.
- See Lower Extremity Stretching Program and Ankle Program. Beware of excessive stretching in the early rehabilitation period.

4. Support

- Wrap the Achilles area and the calf with an elastic bandage or tape.
- The main support is a proper shoe with a stable heel.

5. Thermal Treatment

- Local ice massage to reduce inflammation.
- Heat before and after activity to loosen muscles.

6. Medication

- Take simple anti-inflammatory medication in the form of ibuprofen or aspirin.
- Local steroid injection is sometimes called for in the tendon sheath, but not directly into the tendon.

7. Equipment

- A very stable running shoe with an elevated heel to reduce the pressure on the heel.
- Simple orthotics (arch supports) in the shoe to control pronation. Custom-made orthotics helpful in some cases.

8. Nutrition

- Avoid obesity. A low-fat, high-carbohydrate diet is very helpful.

9. Fluids

- Maintain fluid intake during exercise to prevent fatigue and muscle dehydration.

10. Surfaces

- Avoid steep inclines and hills.
- Stay on soft surfaces such as blacktop and asphalt biking paths.

36. Torn Achilles Tendon

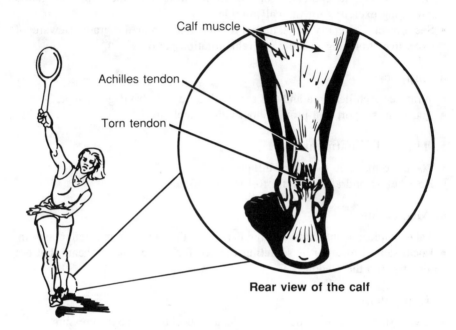

Calf muscle

Achilles tendon

Torn tendon

Rear view of the calf

6-POINT CONDITION SUMMARY

Definition

A traumatic tendon condition characterized by a total disruption of the large tendon behind the ankle (Achilles tendon) and resulting in acute pain and inability to walk.

Cause

- A slow, gradual deterioration or degeneration of the tendon.
- An acute, sudden overload causing total disruption of the fibers.
- In a middle-aged person, an overloading on the Achilles tendon. Possibly also associated with foot imbalance.

Subjective Symptoms

- Gradual pain behind the ankle leading to explosive and intense pain and a sharp sensation as if you were kicked or hit.
- Total inability to walk on the toes.
- Progressive swelling.

Objective Findings

- There is well-localized tenderness and a gap in the Achilles tendon.
- Squeezing the calf (Thompson's test) produces no plantar flexion of the ankle.
- Neurologic exam is normal.

Testing Procedures

- Routine X-rays are negative, but a small spur may appear.
- Degenerative changes may be present in the bone.
- Arthrogram is not helpful.
- MRI may show disruption of the tendon.

Prognosis

Many philosophies of treatment are available. Some surgeons recommend immediate surgery. Some recommend casting for 2 to 3 months. Six to 9 months of healing may be required before returning to jumping activities. This injury may threaten careers in sports that require jumping such as basketball or football.

10-POINT TREATMENT PLAN

1. Activity Levels

- During casting, biking with the well leg, walking, and upper-body aerobic conditioning and weight lifting are indicated.

2. Alternative Activities

- Running in a swimming pool with a plastic bag over the cast.
- Biking with the well leg.
- Upper-body rowing.

3. Rehab Exercises

- Rest is required—no running or jumping.
- Do upper-body exercises during casting.
- See Lower Extremity Stretching Program and Ankle Program. Beware of excessive stretching in early rehabilitation period.

4. Support

- Cast is indicated for many months, followed by an air-bag ankle splint.
- Progress to simple elastic ankle wraps and a heel lift.

5. Thermal Treatment

- Ice massage initially to reduce pain and swelling.
- Local heat to the calf to reduce muscle soreness.

6. Medication

- Take simple anti-inflammatory medication along with stronger codeine medications.
- Avoid steroid injections.

7. Equipment

- Initially, a cast is required with the foot in plantar flexion (toes down), whether or not you have surgery.
- Use Aerodyne bike for upper-body exercise.

8. Nutrition

- During periods of immobilization, avoid obesity with a low-fat, high-carbohydrate diet.

9. Fluids

- Maintain good hydration during periods of training to maintain muscle function.

10. Surfaces

- Avoid exercising on hills and performing twisting activities.
- When cast is removed and rehabilitation has progressed appropriately, run on soft surfaces such as blacktop or bicycle paths.

37. Lateral Ligament Sprain

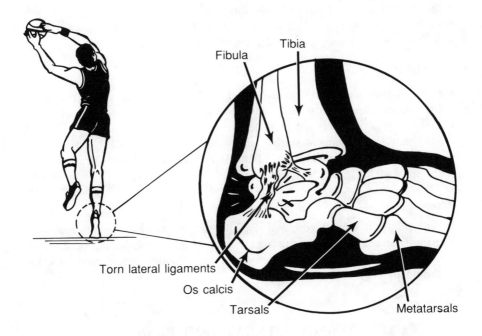

Fibula | Tibia

Torn lateral ligaments
Os calcis
Tarsals | Metatarsals

6-POINT CONDITION SUMMARY

Definition

A traumatic ankle injury, associated with a twisting injury to the outer (lateral) ligaments. Associated with acute pain, swelling, and limp.

Cause

- Acute: a sudden twisting or inversion (an inward tilting) of the ankle.
- Chronic: repetitive ankle sprains with progressive stretching and tearing of the ligaments. May lead to chronic recurrent instability.

Subjective Symptoms

- Pain well localized to the outer tip of the ankle bone.
- Swelling occurs within a few hours.
- A sensation of giving way present with repeated sprains.
- Crepitation generally not present.

Objective Findings

- Tenderness is well localized to the outer tip of the ankle bone.
- Swelling is present from local bleeding.
- Instability: Ligament testing will reveal the ankle is giving way.
- Stiffness and loss of motion are present because of swelling and pain.

Testing Procedures

- Initial X-rays are usually normal but may show associated small fractures.
- Chronic cases may show bone spurs and loose fragments on stress X-rays.
- Bone scan generally is not indicated.
- MRI may show ligament tearing.
- Arthroscopy is generally not indicated but may reveal bony fragments in chronic cases.

Prognosis

With proper treatment, rest, and rehabilitation, acute cases usually heal with a resulting stable ankle. Chronic, recurrent tears in a loose-jointed person may lead to a chronically unstable ankle, which may require surgical reconstruction of the ligaments.

10-POINT TREATMENT PLAN

1. Activity Levels

- During initial splinting and casting, let pain be the guide.
- Maintain general aerobic conditioning and upper-body strength.

2. Alternative Activities

- Swimming and running in a pool may be advisable with the permission of a physician.
- A plastic bag can be put over the ankle if cast is used.
- Upper-body aerobic conditioning and weight lifting are permissible.

3. Rehab Exercises

- During casting, continue isometric ankle and knee exercises.
- During rehabilitation, work on flexibility and strength with weights and tubing.
- See Lower Extremity Strengthening Program and Ankle Program.

4. Support

- Acute cases may need tape, splints, or a cast.
- Chronic cases during rehabilitation may need air stirrup splints.

5. Thermal Treatment

- Apply ice locally for the first 2 or 3 days.
- Avoid heat if any unusual swelling is present.

6. Medication

- During the first 2 or 3 days, codeine may be required.
- Chronic cases may need aspirin or ibuprofen.

7. Equipment

- Wear hightop shoes with extremely stable heels.

8. Nutrition

- Maintain low body fat with a high-carbohydrate, low-fat diet.

9. Fluids

- Maintain good hydration.

10. Surfaces

- Be very careful when running on uneven ground and terrain.
- Avoid running on extremely firm surfaces such as cement streets.

38. Metatarsal Stress Fracture

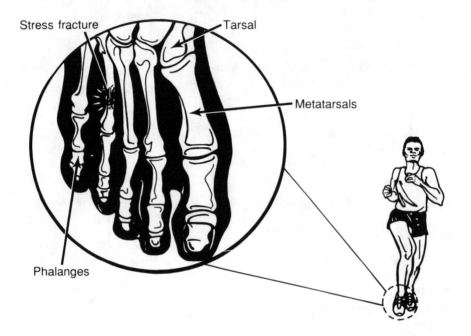

Stress fracture — Tarsal

Metatarsals

Phalanges

6-POINT CONDITION SUMMARY

Definition

An overuse condition in the bone, characterized by a microfracture of the metatarsal bone. An aching pain in the foot during long running.

Cause

- Acute: a sudden pain or snap in a previously weakened bone. Occurs during a jump.
- Chronic: repeated microtrauma in a runner or dancer with foot imbalance who performs on hard surfaces. Associated factors: obesity, malnutrition, and, in some cases, eating disorders.

Subjective Symptoms

- Pain well localized directly over the bone on top of the foot.
- Swelling initially not present.
- Stiffness present after running.
- Crepitation not present.

Metatarsal Stress Fracture

Objective Findings

- Tenderness is well localized to the bone surface.
- Local swelling may be present as the healing bone forms.
- Loss of motion is not present.

Testing Procedures

- Initial X-rays may be normal, but X-rays 2 or 3 weeks later will show healing bone formation.
- Bone scan will be very diagnostic.
- MRI is not required.

Prognosis

The most important aspect of this condition is proper recognition and diagnosis, otherwise many months of bone healing will be required. Total rest is not required. Casting generally is not needed. Many alternative activities are available. Proper shoes and orthotics are very helpful. Avoiding obesity and malnutrition is important.

 10-POINT TREATMENT PLAN

1. Activity Levels

- Reducing intensity of sports is important, but there is no need to stop all activity. Let pain be the guide.
- Displacement of the fracture and surgery are very unusual with moderate activity.

2. Alternative Activities

- Running in water, biking, and swimming are acceptable.

3. Rehab Exercises

- Maintain flexibility, endurance, speed, and strength of the muscles and joints above and below the fracture.
- See Lower Extremity Strengthening Program and Ankle Program.

4. Support

- Casting is rarely indicated, unless pain and swelling are severe.
- Simple protective activities and a good supporting shoe are enough to protect the bone.

5. Thermal Treatment

- Ice massage helps to reduce pain and swelling.

6. Medication

- Avoid medication that may mask the pain and prevent a proper diagnosis.
- Calcium and vitamins are suggested if an eating disorder is present.

7. Equipment

- Proper shoes with good heel control.
- Orthotics (arch supports) for pronated foot.

8. Nutrition

- Evaluate any causes of malnutrition or obesity.
- During rehabilitation, maintain a high-carbohydrate, low-fat diet to avoid obesity.

9. Fluids

- Maintain good hydration.

10. Surfaces

- It is very important to avoid running on concrete or any roughened surfaces that cause excessive impact to the foot.

39. Morton's Neuroma

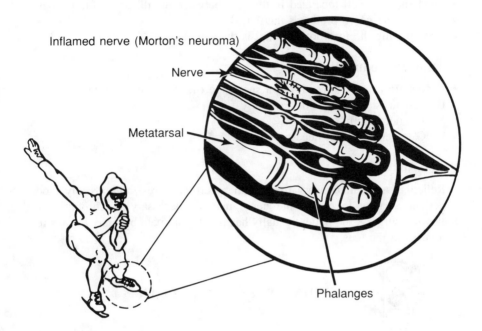

Inflamed nerve (Morton's neuroma)

Nerve

Metatarsal

Phalanges

6-POINT CONDITION SUMMARY

Definition

A traumatic nerve compression of the foot characterized by numbness of the third and fourth toes. Associated with tight shoes and pronated (weak arch) foot.

Cause

- Acute: direct injury to the top of the foot, with resulting swelling and compression of the nerve.
- Chronic: microtrauma to the nerve between the third and fourth toes. May result from a "Morton foot" (a short first toe and a pronated foot).

Subjective Symptoms

- Pain between the third and fourth toes, radiating to the foot.
- Swelling generally not present.
- Limp present while athlete wears tight high-heeled shoes.

Objective Findings

- Tenderness is well localized in the web between the third and fourth toes.
- Pinching the nerve produces numbness.
- Compressing the forefoot reproduces the symptoms.

Testing Procedures

- X-rays are usually normal, but a shortened first toe may be noted.
- Bone scan is generally not necessary.
- MRI is not helpful.
- EMG is generally not necessary.

Prognosis

Relief is usual with conservative treatment: orthotics, rest, and possibly a local injection. Surgery to excise the nerve may be necessary in chronic cases. Following surgery, the patient usually has relief from pain but may always feel numbness in the toes.

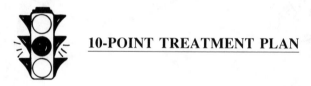 **10-POINT TREATMENT PLAN**

1. Activity Levels

- Continue activities such as running and biking, but with moderation.

2. Alternative Activities

- Stress upper-body weight lifting and biking.

3. Rehab Exercises

- Let pain be the guide.
- Reduce intensity of running and biking, but there is no need to stop.
- See Lower Extremity Strengthening Program and Ankle Program.

4. Support

- A metatarsal bar on the shoe and an orthotic for the arch are helpful.

5. Thermal Treatment

- Local ice massage to reduce pain and swelling.

6. Medication

- Take simple anti-inflammatory medications such as aspirin and ibuprofen.
- Local steroid injection around the nerve may be helpful.

7. Equipment

- Shoes should be wide and have ample room for the toes.
- Be careful of tight toe clips on bicycles.

8. Nutrition

- Follow a high-carbohydrate, low-fat diet.

9. Fluids

- Maintain good hydration.

10. Surfaces

- Beware of hard impact on rough surfaces and concrete.

40. Plantar Fasciitis (Heel Pain)

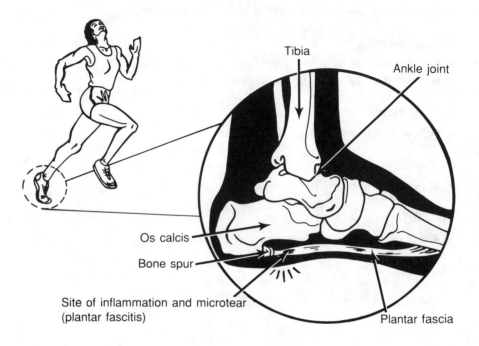

Tibia

Ankle joint

Os calcis

Bone spur

Site of inflammation and microtear
(plantar fascitis)

Plantar fascia

6-POINT CONDITION SUMMARY

Definition

A traumatic, degenerative process characterized by pain along the inner aspect of the heel and radiating along the arch. May occur in a young runner or a middle-aged worker with foot imbalance.

Cause

- Acute: violent jumping and tearing of the plantar fascia (the heavy ligament band along the arch).
- Chronic: microtrauma or overuse of the foot, associated with foot imbalance, muscle imbalance, and tight ligaments in the foot.

Subjective Symptoms

- Pain, especially on awakening in the morning and with first steps.
- Swelling generally not present.

Plantar Fasciitis (Heel Pain)

- Stiffness present, especially in the morning when weight bears down on the rested foot.
- Occasional numbness in the heel.

Objective Findings

- Tenderness is well localized to the inner aspect of the heel.
- Swelling is generally not present.
- Instability of the foot may be present with a pronated foot.
- Nerve exam is generally normal.

Testing Procedures

- X-rays may be normal, but a spur on the heel may be present.
- Scan may show a positive area on the bone where the ligament attaches.
- MRI is generally not necessary.
- Arthroscopy is not done.

Prognosis

Chronic pain due to poor healing is usual because of poor circulation to the ligament and stresses to the heel. Referral to a sports podiatrist to fabricate orthotics may be necessary. Surgery is unusual, but chronic cases may require cutting the ligament where it attaches to the heel.

 ## 10-POINT TREATMENT PLAN

1. Activity Levels

- Continue with moderate running, biking, and jumping, but avoid extremes.

2. Alternative Activities

- Biking and swimming are excellent alternatives during rehabilitation.

3. Rehab Exercises

- Maintain foot flexibility and strength with tubing and simple weights.
- See Lower Extremity Strengthening Program and Ankle Program.

4. Support

- Orthotic device in the shoe to support the arch is helpful.

5. Thermal Treatment

- Local ice massage to the painful area.
- Heat to relieve muscle spasm and tightness.

6. Medication

- Take simple anti-inflammatory medications such as aspirin and ibuprofen.
- Chronic cases may require a prescription for nonsteroidal anti-inflammatory medication.
- Local injection of steroid may be helpful in chronic cases.

7. Equipment

- Use a good, firm-heeled shoe that supports the arch.

8. Nutrition

- Follow a high-carbohydrate, low-fat diet.

9. Fluids

- Maintain good hydration.

10. Surfaces

- Avoid excessive running on hard surfaces such as concrete.
- Avoid running on curves.

PART IV

SPECIFIC REHABILITATION EXERCISE PROGRAMS

The following 15 exercise programs (cross-referenced within Part III) are examples of effective groups of exercises that you can use to help build strength, endurance, flexibility, or speed, depending on your needs:

- Back Flexion Program (see p. 168)
- Back Strengthening Program (see p. 170)
- Beginning Shoulder Program (see p. 173)
- Shoulder Dislocation Program (see p. 176)
- Shoulder Acromioclavicular Program (see p. 180)
- Rotator Cuff Program (see p. 184)
- Upper Extremity Stretching Program (see p. 188)
- Beginning Tennis Elbow Program (see p. 189)
- Advanced Tennis Elbow Program (see p. 191)
- Lower Extremity Stretching Program (see p. 194)
- Lower Extremity Strengthening Program (see p. 197)
- Patellar Program (see p. 199)
- Meniscus Knee Program (see p. 201)
- Anterior Cruciate Knee Program (see p. 204)
- Ankle Program (see p. 207)

These exercise programs are standard, balanced programs used by the physicians, physical therapists, and trainers for athletic rehabilitation of the Sinai Samaritan Medical Center's Sports Medicine Institute, Milwaukee, WI (copyright 1989, adapted with permission). Some exercises direct you to "perform ____ sets, ____ repetitions, ____ times/day." Ask your physical therapist, trainer, coach, or health care provider for guidance in determining how many sets and repetitions to perform each day.

All strengthening exercises require simple home techniques using 5-pound sandbags and exercise tubing. Exercise tubing can be purchased from athletic supply stores. If tubing is not available, a rubber bicycle inner tube is suggested.

With all stretching exercises, remember that the best time to stretch a muscle is when it is warm. Therefore, always precede any stretching program with activities that will increase your blood's circulation, such as slowly marching, jogging, or walking. Then, stretch slowly and hold the stretch position for 20 to 30 seconds, without bouncing. Repeat at least three times. Another excellent time to stretch is at the end of a practice or work-out—when you are already warm and "loose."

• BACK FLEXION PROGRAM •

During the acute painful phase of many back problems, the flexed position and flexion exercises may be helpful to relieve pressure on discs and nerves. Avoid any position or activity which may increase pain or radiation of discomfort down your leg. Let your therapist or physician know if you have any question or increase in pain with the exercises.

PELVIC TILTS

1. Lie on back with knees bent and feet flat on floor.
2. Tighten stomach and buttock muscles.
3. "Rock" pelvis backward, pushing small of back against floor.
4. Hold for 5 seconds and relax.

a

b

PELVIC CLOCK

1. Lie on back on floor with knees bent and feet flat on floor.
2. Picture a clock on your stomach and tilt pelvis toward each number.

KNEES TO CHEST

1. Lie on back with knees bent.
2. Lift left knee, and with aid of arms, pull knee gently toward chest until stretch is felt in lower back.

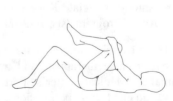

3. Hold 5 seconds.
4. Return leg to starting position and relax.
5. Repeat with right leg.
6. Perform ＿＿ sets, ＿＿ repetitions, ＿＿ times/day.

BOTH KNEES TO CHEST

1. Lie on back with knees bent.
2. Lift both knees to chest, one at a time with aid of arms until stretch is felt in lower back.
3. Hold 5 seconds.
4. Perform ＿＿ sets, ＿＿ repetitions, ＿＿ times/day.

PARTIAL SIT-UPS

1. Lie on back with knees bent and feet flat on floor. (Perform a pelvic tilt.)
2. Tuck chin and raise shoulder blades off floor, reaching with arms straight toward knees.
3. Lower shoulders and arms to floor (and release pelvic tilt).
4. Relax.
5. Repeat, rotating first to the right and then to the left.
6. Perform ＿＿ sets, ＿＿ repetitions, ＿＿ times/day.

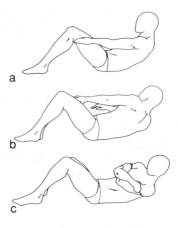

PELVIC ROTATIONS

1. Lie on back with knees bent and feet flat on floor.
2. Keep knees together and rock legs to the left until a moderate stretch is noted. Hold for 5 seconds.
3. Return to starting position and repeat to the right.
4. Perform ＿＿ sets, ＿＿ repetitions, ＿＿ times/day.

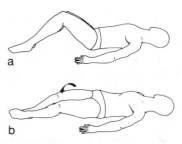

• BACK STRENGTHENING PROGRAM •

Lumbar and thoracic back strength is provided mainly by the extensor (back) muscle groups. As pain subsides and pressure is off of the nerve, progressive extension or straightening exercises are helpful when approved by your physician. Avoid any motion or exercise that may increase pain.

PRONE ON ELBOWS

1. Lie on stomach on floor or bed.
2. Raise or prop up on both elbows, allowing back to sag and form an arch.
3. Hold for 10 seconds and return to starting position.

PRONE PRESS-UPS

1. Lie on stomach with hands at shoulders.
2. Slowly straighten arms and press up, keeping hips down on flat surface.
3. Hold position for 10 seconds.
4. Return to starting position.

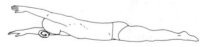

ALTERNATE ARM LIFTS

1. Lie on stomach with arms raised above head, legs straight.
2. Slowly tighten left hand, forearm, and shoulder musculature.
3. Raise arm 3 or more inches off floor.
4. Hold 5 to 10 seconds.
5. Slowly lower arm to floor.
6. Repeat sequence with right arm.

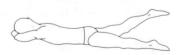

ALTERNATE LEG LIFTS

1. Lie on stomach with legs straight, arms crossed above head.
2. Rest head on arms and turn head either right or left.
3. Slowly tighten right buttock and thigh musculature.
4. Raise right leg approximately 3 inches off floor.

5. Hold 5 to 10 seconds.
6. Slowly lower leg to floor.
7. Repeat above sequence with left leg.

EXTENSION TO NEUTRAL
(CHEST LIFTS)

1. Place one or two pillows under stomach and hips. Lie face down with arms at sides.
2. Raise head, trunk, and chest off floor to a horizontal position.
3. Hold 5 seconds and slowly lower trunk, chest, and head to floor and relax.

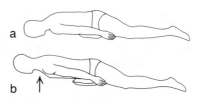

ALTERNATE ARM
AND LEG LIFTS

1. Lie on stomach with towel roll under forehead, arms straight and overhead.
2. Slowly tighten left arm and right leg.
3. Raise arm and leg approximately 3 inches toward ceiling.
4. Hold 5 seconds.
5. Slowly lower left arm and right leg to floor.
6. Repeat entire sequence with right arm and left leg.

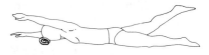

BILATERAL ARM LIFTS

1. Lie on stomach with towel roll under forehead, legs straight and arms overhead and straight.
2. Slowly tighten hands, forearms, and shoulders.
3. Slowly raise arms off floor approximately 3 inches.
4. Hold 5 to 10 seconds.
5. Slowly lower arms to floor.

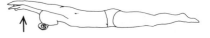

HANDS AND KNEES

1. Support yourself evenly on your hands and knees, head and eyes looking toward the floor.
2. Slowly tighten left arm and right leg.
3. Raise left arm and right leg off floor to horizontal position.
4. Hold 5 seconds.
5. Slowly lower arm and leg to floor.
6. Repeat above sequence with right arm and left leg.

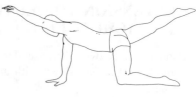

BRIDGING

1. Lie on back with knees bent and slightly apart, feet flat on floor.
2. Tighten buttock muscles.
3. Raise buttocks off floor until level with knees.
4. Hold for 5 seconds.
5. Slowly lower buttocks to floor.

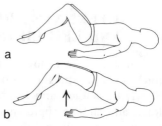

CAT EXERCISE

1. Begin on hands and knees.
2. Drop chin and arch back like a cat.
3. Hold 5 seconds.
4. Relax and allow back to sag.
5. Repeat.

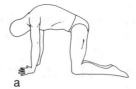

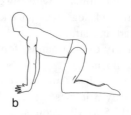

● BEGINNING SHOULDER PROGRAM ●

The shoulder joint, being very flexible, can scar and tighten very easily. This is called a "frozen shoulder." Regardless of your shoulder condition, it is important to start early motion when approved by your physician and therapist.

CODMAN'S

1. Lean on a table with your uninvolved elbow bent 90 degrees.
2. Let your involved arm hang straight down, and use your body to initiate a pendular swinging motion.
3. Move your arm (a) side to side, (b) forward and back, and (c) in circles clockwise and counterclockwise.
4. *DO NOT* swing your arm.

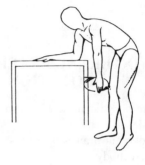

CANE EXERCISES

Flexion

1. Lie on your back with knees bent and cane in both hands.
2. Raise cane slowly over your head as far as possible.
3. Return to starting position.
4. Perform ___ sets, ___ repetitions, ___ times/day.

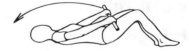

Horizontal Abduction

1. Lie on your back, cane in both hands.
2. Bring cane up to 90 degrees, then bring as far to the left as possible, then as far to the right as possible.
3. Return to starting position.
4. Perform ___ sets, ___ repetitions, ___ times/day.

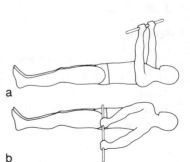

a

b

Abduction

1. Sit or stand with cane in both hands, involved palm upward.
2. Push cane out to the side as far as possible.
3. Return to starting position.
4. Perform ___ sets, ___ repetitions, ___ times/day.

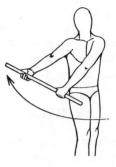

INTERNAL/EXTERNAL ROTATION

1. Lie on your back with arm by your side.
2. Rotate arm away from body, then in toward body.
3. Gradually progress moving arm out to 90 degrees from side of body.
4. Perform ___ sets, ___ repetitions, ___ times/day.

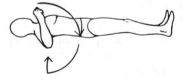

ISOMETRICS

Flexion

1. Sit with involved arm by side of body.
2. With opposite hand, resist forward movement of arm, holding for five counts.
3. Relax.
4. Perform ___ sets, ___ repetitions, ___ times/day.

Extension

1. Sit with arm by side of body in flexed position.
2. With opposite hand, resist backward movement of arm, holding for five counts.
3. Relax.
4. Perform ___ sets, ___ repetitions, ___ times/day.

Abduction

1. Sit with arm by side of body in flexed position.
2. With opposite hand, resist sideways movement of arm, holding for five counts.
3. Perform ____ sets, ____ repetitions, ____ times/day.

External Rotation

1. Stand with outer side of injured arm against doorjamb, elbow bent 90 degrees and held close to body.
2. Try to push hard outward against doorjamb, holding for five counts.
3. Perform ____ sets, ____ repetitions, ____ times/day.

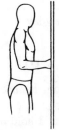

Internal Rotation

1. Stand with inner side of injured arm against doorjamb, elbow bent 90 degrees and held close to body.
2. Try to push inward against doorjamb, holding for five counts.
3. Perform ____ sets, ____ repetitions, ____ times/day.

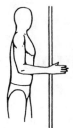

SHOULDER SHRUGS

1. Sit or stand in an upright position with shoulders back and arms at sides.
2. Place weight over top of shoulder or in hand as directed by your therapist.
3. Slowly raise or shrug shoulders up to ears.
4. Hold for 5 seconds.
5. Slowly lower to starting position.
6. Perform ____ sets, ____ repetitions, ____ times/day.

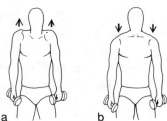

a   b

SHOULDER PROTRACTION/ RETRACTION

1. Rest arm on table at about shoulder level.
2. Reach arm forward as far as possible, then pull back as far as possible.
3. Perform ____ sets, ____ repetitions, ____ times/day.

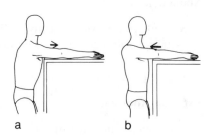

a   b

WEIGHT SHIFTING

1. Lie on your stomach propped on both elbows.
2. Lean to one side and hold position for a few seconds, then move to opposite side and hold a few seconds.
3. Repeat.

● SHOULDER DISLOCATION PROGRAM ●

Shoulder dislocation or subluxation occurs when the ligaments surrounding your shoulder joint are stretched or torn. To improve the stability in your shoulder, special strengthening exercises are necessary. Please let your therapist know if you have any questions or an increase in pain with the exercises.

INTERNAL ROTATION

1. Place tubing in door at elbow level.
2. Stand sideways to door with your injured arm toward the door.
3. Bend elbow 90 degrees and place small towel roll between arm and body.
4. Grasp tubing and rotate it in toward your opposite hip.
5. Slowly return to starting position.
6. Perform ____ sets, ____ repetitions, ____ times/day.

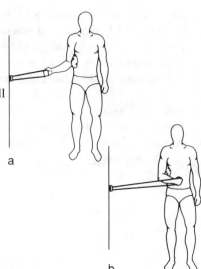

a

b

ADDUCTION

1. Tie tubing to doorknob.
2. Stand with involved arm toward door.
3. Hold tubing in hand and pull directly across body.
4. Return to starting position.
5. Perform ____ sets, ____ repetitions, ____ times/day.

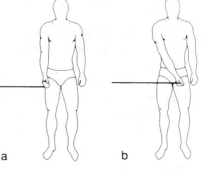

a   b

EXTENSION

Standing

1. Place tubing in door at elbow level.
2. With injured arm down at your side, grasp tubing and pull it directly behind you.
3. Do not bend forward at the waist while pulling back.
4. Slowly return to starting position.
5. Perform ____ sets, ____ repetitions, ____ times/day.

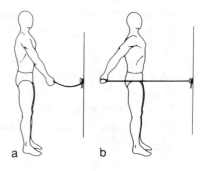

a   b

Lying Prone

1. Lie on your stomach, with injured arm hanging over side of bed or couch.
2. Tie tubing directly below or near hand level.
3. Grasp tubing and pull arm up along side of body.
4. Slowly return to starting position.
5. Perform ____ sets, ____ repetitions, ____ times/day.

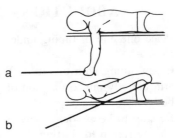

a

b

FLEXION

1. Place one end of tubing under your foot.
2. Grasp tubing with thumb on top, and lift arm directly out to the front of your body.
3. Be sure to keep your elbow straight.
4. Slowly return to starting position.
5. Perform ____ sets, ____ repetitions, ____ times/day.

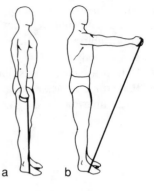

a   b

HORIZONTAL ABDUCTION

1. Lie on your stomach with your injured arm over the side of bed or couch.
2. Tie tubing directly below shoulder level.
3. Grasp tubing and pull straight out from your body 90 degrees at shoulder height.
4. Slowly return to starting position.
5. Perform ____ sets, ____ repetitions, ____ times/day.

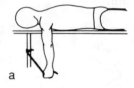

a

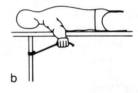

b

ABDUCTION

1. Place one end of tubing under your foot.
2. Grasp tubing with thumb on top and lift arm directly out to the side of your body.
3. Be sure to keep your elbow straight.
4. Slowly return to starting position.
5. Perform ____ sets, ____ repetitions, ____ times/day.

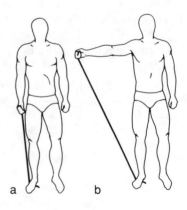

a   b

EMPTY CAN

1. Place middle of tubing under your feet.
2. Grasp tubing in both hands with thumbs turned down.
3. Rather than lifting your arms straight out to the side, raise your arms in a position 30 degrees forward of that position.
4. Keep elbows straight and *do not* lift above shoulder level.
5. Slowly return to original position.
6. Perform ____ sets, ____ repetitions, ____ times/day.

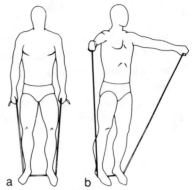

EXTERNAL ROTATION

1. Hold tubing in both hands.
2. Anchor hand of uninjured arm on hip.
3. Bend elbow of injured arm 90 degrees, and place small towel roll in between arm and body.
4. Grasp tubing and rotate it out away from your body.
5. Slowly return to starting position.
6. Perform ____ sets, ____ repetitions, ____ times/day.

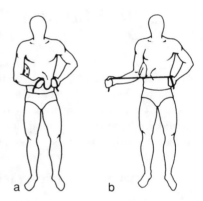

HORIZONTAL PULL

1. Hold tubing in both hands at shoulder height.
2. Pull tubing apart until arms are directly out to each side of your body.
3. Slowly return to starting position.
4. Perform ____ sets, ____ repetitions, ____ times/day.

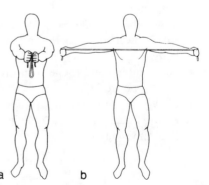

DIAGONAL PULL

1. Hold tubing in both hands at shoulder height.
2. Pull tubing apart at a diagonal with injured arm angled above shoulder height and uninjured arm angled below shoulder height.
3. Slowly return to starting position.
4. Perform ___ sets, ___ repetitions, ___ times/day.

a   b

• SHOULDER ACROMIOCLAVICULAR • PROGRAM

Acromioclavicular (AC) joint sprain is a stretching or tearing of the ligaments on the top joint of the shoulder. If you have an injury in this joint, special exercises are necessary to increase your muscle strength and stabilize your shoulder. Please let your therapist know if you have any questions or an increase in pain with the exercises.

INTERNAL ROTATION

1. Place tubing in door at elbow level.
2. Stand sideways to door with your injured arm toward the door.
3. Bend elbow 90 degrees, and place small towel roll in between arm and body.
4. Grasp tubing and rotate it in toward your opposite hip.
5. Slowly return to starting position.
6. Perform ___ sets, ___ repetitions, ___ times/day.

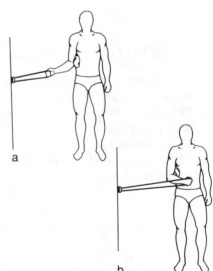

a

b

EXTERNAL ROTATION

1. Hold tubing in both hands.
2. Anchor hand of uninjured arm on hip.
3. Bend elbow of injured arm 90 degrees, and place small towel roll in between arm and body.
4. Grasp tubing and rotate it out, away from your body.
5. Slowly return to starting position.
6. Perform ____ sets, ____ repetitions, ____ times/day.

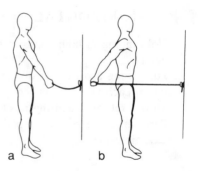

a   b

EXTENSION

Standing

1. Place tubing in door at elbow level.
2. With injured arm down at your side, grasp tubing and pull it directly behind you.
3. Do not bend forward at the waist while pulling back.
4. Slowly return to starting position.
5. Perform ____ sets, ____ repetitions, ____ times/day.

a   b

Lying Prone

1. Lie on your stomach, with injured arm hanging over side of bed or couch.
2. Tie tubing directly below or near hand level.
3. Grasp tubing and pull arm up along side of body.
4. Slowly return to starting position.
5. Perform ____ sets, ____ repetitions, ____ times/day.

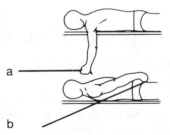

a

b

HORIZONTAL ABDUCTION

1. Lie on your stomach with your injured arm over the side of your bed or couch.
2. Tie tubing directly below shoulder level.
3. Grasp tubing and pull straight out from your body 90 degrees at shoulder height.
4. Slowly return to starting position.
5. Perform _____ sets, _____ repetitions, _____ times/day.

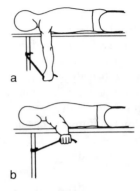

HORIZONTAL PULL

1. Hold tubing in both hands at shoulder height.
2. Pull tubing apart until arms are directly out to each side of your body.
3. Slowly return to starting position.
4. Perform _____ sets, _____ repetitions, _____ times/day.

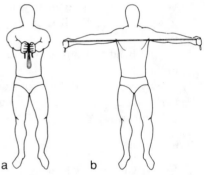

DIAGONAL PULL

1. Hold tubing in both hands at shoulder height.
2. Pull tubing apart at a diagonal with injured arm angled below shoulder height and uninjured arm angled above shoulder height.
3. Slowly return to starting position.
4. Perform _____ sets, _____ repetitions, _____ times/day.

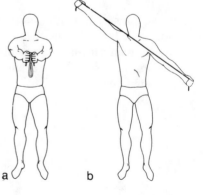

FLEXION

1. Place one end of tubing under your foot.
2. Grasp tubing with thumb on top, and lift arm directly out to the front of your body.
3. Be sure to keep your elbow straight.
4. Slowly return to starting position.
5. Perform ____ sets, ____ repetitions, ____ times/day.

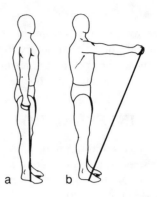

ABDUCTION

1. Place one end of tubing under your foot.
2. Grasp tubing with thumb on top, and lift arm directly out to the side of your body.
3. Be sure to keep your elbow straight.
4. Slowly return to starting position.
5. Perform ____ sets, ____ repetitions, ____ times/day.

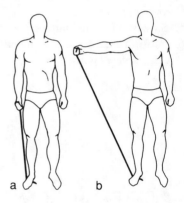

SHOULDER SHRUGS

1. Sit or stand in an upright posture with shoulders back and arms at sides.
2. Place weight over top of shoulder or in hand as directed by your therapist.
3. Slowly raise or shrug shoulders up to ears.
4. Hold for 5 seconds.
5. Slowly lower to starting position.
6. Perform ____ sets, ____ repetitions, ____ times/day.

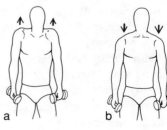

● ROTATOR CUFF PROGRAM ●

The rotator cuff is a group of four muscles/tendons which move the shoulder joint. If you have an injury to your rotator cuff, special strengthening exercises are necessary before you resume normal activity. Please let your therapist know if you have any questions or an increase in pain with the exercises.

INTERNAL ROTATION

1. Place tubing in door at elbow level.
2. Stand sideways to door with your injured arm toward the door.
3. Bend elbow 90 degrees, and place small towel roll between arm and body.
4. Grasp tubing and rotate it in toward your opposite hip.
5. Slowly return to starting position.
6. Perform ____ sets, ____ repetitions, ____ times/day.

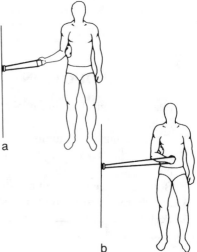

EXTERNAL ROTATION

1. Hold tubing in both hands.
2. Anchor hand of uninjured arm on hip.
3. Bend elbow of injured arm 90 degrees, and place small towel roll in between arm and body.
4. Grasp tubing and rotate it out, away from your body.
5. Slowly return to starting position.
6. Perform ____ sets, ____ repetitions, ____ times/day.

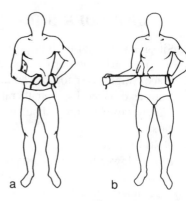

EXTENSION

Standing

1. Place tubing in door at elbow level.
2. With injured arm down at your side, grasp tubing and pull it directly behind you.
3. Do not bend forward at the waist while pulling back.
4. Slowly return to starting position.
5. Perform ____ sets, ____ repetitions, ____ times/day.

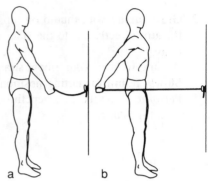

Lying Prone

1. Lie on your stomach, with injured arm hanging over side of bed or couch.
2. Tie tubing directly below or near hand level.
3. Grasp tubing and pull arm up along side of body.
4. Slowly return to starting position.
5. Perform ____ sets, ____ repetitions, ____ times/day.

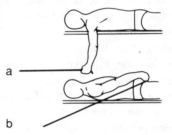

FLEXION

1. Place one end of tubing under your foot.
2. Grasp tubing with thumb on top, and lift arm directly out to the front of your body.
3. Be sure to keep your elbow straight.
4. Slowly return to starting position.
5. Perform ____ sets, ____ repetitions, ____ times/day.

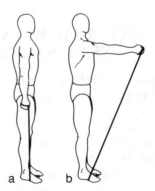

ABDUCTION

1. Place one end of tubing under your foot.
2. Grasp tubing with thumb on top, and lift arm directly out to the side of your body.
3. Be sure to keep your elbow straight.
4. Slowly return to starting position.
5. Perform ___ sets, ___ repetitions, ___ times/day.

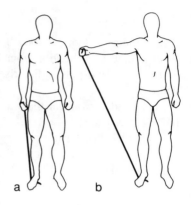

EMPTY CAN

1. Place middle of tubing under your feet.
2. Grasp tubing in both hands with thumbs turned down.
3. Rather than lifting your arms straight out to the side, raise your arms in a position 30 degrees forward of that position.
4. Keep elbows straight and *do not* lift above shoulder level.
5. Slowly return to starting position.
6. Perform ___ sets, ___ repetitions, ___ times/day.

EXTERNAL ROTATION AT 90 DEGREES

1. Lie on your back on a firm surface.
2. Place one end of tubing around your foot.
3. Raise arm out to side (90 degrees) shoulder height, and bend your elbow up 90 degrees.
4. Grasp tubing and rotate backward until the back of your hand hits the firm surface.
5. Slowly return to starting position.
6. Perform ___ sets, ___ repetitions, ___ times/day.

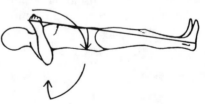

HORIZONTAL ABDUCTION

1. Lie on your stomach with your injured arm over the side of your bed or couch.
2. Tie tubing directly below shoulder level.
3. Grasp tubing and pull straight out from your body 90 degrees at shoulder height.
4. Slowly return to starting position.
5. Perform ____ sets, ____ repetitions, ____ times/day.

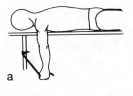
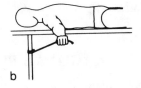

PRONE ON ELBOWS WITH EXTERNAL ROTATION

1. Lie on your stomach, propped up on your elbows.
2. Hold tubing in both hands about shoulder-width apart.
3. Try to pull tubing apart and hold 5 seconds.
4. Slowly return to starting position.
5. Perform ____ sets, ____ repetitions, ____ times/day.

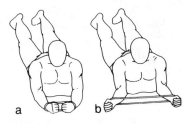

WALL PUSH-UPS

1. Stand arm's length away from the wall.
2. Place hands on wall, with fingers pointing in toward each other.
3. Slowly bend your elbows, bringing your chest in toward the wall. (Elbows should point straight out from your body.)
4. Slowly return to starting position.
5. Perform ____ sets, ____ repetitions, ____ times/day.

HORIZONTAL PULL

1. Hold tubing in both hands at shoulder height.
2. Pull tubing apart until arms are directly out to each side of your body.
3. Slowly return to the starting position.
4. Perform _____ sets, _____ repetitions, _____ times/day.

DIAGONAL PULL

1. Hold tubing in both hands at shoulder height.
2. Pull tubing apart at a diagonal with injured arm angled above shoulder height and uninjured arm angled below shoulder height.
3. Slowly return to starting position.
4. Perform _____ sets, _____ repetitions, _____ times/day.

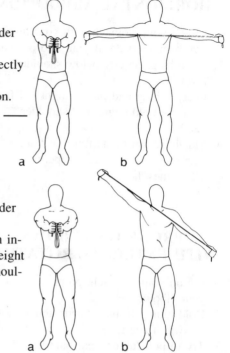

● UPPER EXTREMITY STRETCHING PROGRAM ●

Flexibility exercises are done to increase overall muscle length. This reduces the incidence of injuries such as muscle strains, pulls, or tears. Flexibility exercises also increase efficiency and therefore improve performance. All stretching should be static; NO BOUNCING STRETCHES! Stretching should be slightly uncomfortable but not painful. Do each stretch slowly and hold for 20 to 30 seconds. Repeat three to five times.

Note: Shading indicates area being stretched.

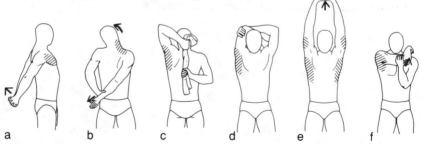

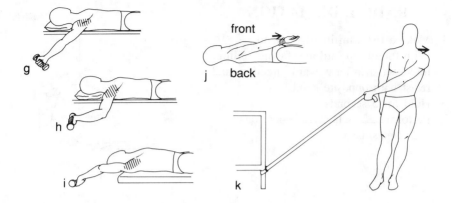

● BEGINNING TENNIS ELBOW PROGRAM ●

Tennis elbow is a commonly used term for inflammation of the tendons on the outside or inside of your elbow. To promote healing and prevent reinjury, you should perform the following exercises as instructed by your therapist. Please let your therapist know if you have any questions or an increase in pain with the exercises.

ISOMETRIC WRIST EXTENSION

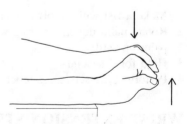

1. Make a fist with involved hand with *palm down*.
2. Move wrist in an upward direction, and resist with opposite hand.
3. Hold for 5 seconds.
4. Perform ____ sets, ____ repetitions, ____ times/day.

WRIST FLEXION

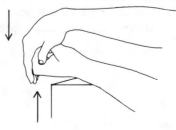

1. Make a fist with involved hand.
2. With *palm up*, move wrist in an upward direction, and resist with opposite hand.
3. Hold for 5 seconds.
4. Perform ____ sets, ____ repetitions, ____ times/day.

RADIAL DEVIATION

1. Make a fist with involved hand.
2. With thumb upward and facing ceiling, move wrist in an upward direction, and resist with opposite hand.
3. Hold for 5 seconds.
4. Perform ___ sets, ___ repetitions, ___ times/day.

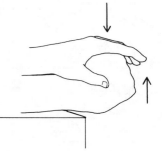

FINGER EXTENSION

1. Make a fist with involved hand, *palm down.*
2. Move fingers from bent into straightened position, resisting with opposite hand.
3. Hold for 5 seconds.
4. Perform ___ sets, ___ repetitions, ___ times/day.

PRONATION/SUPINATION

1. Make a fist with involved hand, with thumb upward and facing ceiling.
2. Rotate palm down, resisting with opposite hand. Repeat while rotating palm upward.
3. Hold for 5 seconds.
4. Perform ___ sets, ___ repetitions, ___ times/day.

WRIST EXTENSION STRETCH

1. Raise arm to shoulder height with elbow straight.
2. Grasp hand and bend down until a mild stretch is felt on the top of arm.
3. Hold 20 to 30 seconds and relax.
4. Perform ___ sets, ___ repetitions, ___ times/day.

WRIST FLEXION STRETCH

1. Raise arm to shoulder height with elbow straight.
2. Grasp hand and bend up until a mild stretch is felt on the bottom of arm.
3. Hold 20 to 30 seconds and relax.
4. Perform ____ sets, ____ repetitions, ____ times/day.

GRIPPING

1. Place a tennis or racquetball in palm of hand.
2. Squeeze and hold for 10 seconds.
3. Perform ____ sets, ____ repetitions, ____ times/day.

● ADVANCED TENNIS ELBOW PROGRAM ●

Tennis elbow is a commonly used term for inflammation of the tendons on the outside or inside of your elbow. To promote healing and prevent reinjury, you should perform the following exercises as instructed by your therapist. Please let your therapist know if you have any questions or an increase in pain with the exercises.

WRIST EXTENSION

1. Sit in a chair with tubing under foot, handle in hand, with palm down. Support forearm on thigh, with wrist and hand extended beyond knee.
2. Slowly raise hand and bend wrist back as far as possible.
3. Slowly return to starting position.
4. Perform ____ sets, ____ repetitions, ____ times/day.

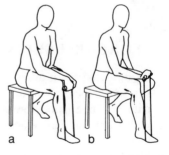

a   b

WRIST FLEXION

1. Sit in a chair with tubing under foot, handle in hand, with palm up. Support forearm on thigh, with wrist and hand extended beyond knee.
2. Slowly curl wrist up as far as possible.
3. Slowly return to starting position.
4. Perform _____ sets, _____ repetitions, _____ times/day.

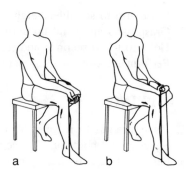

a   b

FOREARM PRONATION

1. Sit in a chair with tubing under foot about 10 inches outside center of body. Hold handle in hand, with palm up. Support forearm on thigh, with wrist and hand extended beyond knee.
2. Slowly rotate forearm to palm down position.
3. Slowly return to starting position.
4. Perform _____ sets, _____ repetitions, _____ times/day.

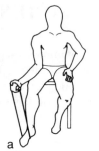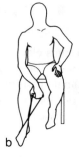

a   b

FOREARM SUPINATION

1. Sit in a chair with tubing under opposite foot. Hold handle in hand, with palm down. Support forearm on thigh, with wrist and hand extended beyond knee.
2. Slowly rotate forearm to palm up position.
3. Slowly return to starting position.
4. Perform _____ sets, _____ repetitions, _____ times/day.

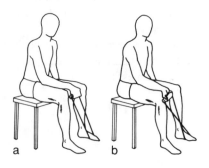

a   b

RADIAL DEVIATION

1. Sit in a chair with tubing under foot. Hold handle in hand, with thumb and handle end pointing up. Support forearm on thigh, with wrist and hand extended beyond knee.
2. Lift hand up toward forearm as high as possible.
3. Slowly return to starting position.
4. Perform ____ sets, ____ repetitions, ____ times/day.

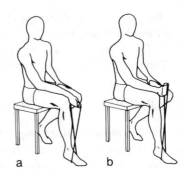

a   b

ELBOW EXTENSION

1. In a standing position, hold tubing in hand. With tubing draped over opposite shoulder, grasp behind back.
2. Straighten elbow raising arm overhead.
3. Slowly return to starting position.
4. Perform ____ sets, ____ repetitions, ____ times/day.

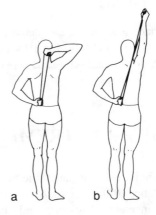

a   b

ELBOW FLEXION

1. Sit in a chair with tubing under foot. Hold handle in hand, palm up. Support elbow on thigh, with forearm, hand, and wrist extended beyond knee.
2. Slowly bend elbow up to a fully flexed position.
3. Slowly return to starting position.
4. Perform ____ sets, ____ repetitions, ____ times/day.

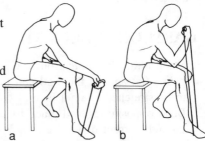

a   b

WRIST EXTENSION STRETCH

1. Raise arm to shoulder height with elbow straight.
2. Grasp hand and bend down until a mild stretch is felt on top of arm.
3. Hold for 20 to 30 seconds and relax.
4. Perform ____ sets, ____ repetitions, ____ times/day.

WRIST FLEXION STRETCH

1. Raise arm to shoulder height with elbow straight.
2. Grasp hand and bend up until a mild stretch is felt on the bottom of arm.
3. Hold for 20 to 30 seconds and relax.
4. Perform ____ sets, ____ repetitions, ____ times/day.

GRIPPING

1. Place a tennis or racquetball in palm of hand.
2. Squeeze and hold for 10 seconds.
3. Perform ____ sets, ____ repetitions, ____ times/day.

●LOWER EXTREMITY STRETCHING PROGRAM ●

Flexibility exercises are done to increase overall muscle length. This reduces the incidence of injuries such as muscle strains, pulls, or tears. Flexibility exercises also increase efficiency and therefore improve performance. All stretching should be static; NO BOUNCING STRETCHES! Stretching should be slightly uncomfortable but not painful. Do each stretch slowly and hold for 20 to 30 seconds. Repeat three to five times.

Note: Arrows indicate the direction of the stretch. Warm up the muscle group you intend to stretch.

GASTROC-SOLEUS STRETCH

1. Stand at arm's length from a wall, palms flat against the wall and the leg to be stretched straight behind you.
2. Bend opposite leg and place foot on the ground in front of you.

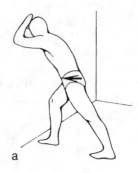

a

3. Keep heel of backward leg down, and keep arch up, toes curled under.
4. Slowly move your hips forward, keeping back straight until a stretch is felt in back of calf.
5. Hold 20 to 30 seconds. Repeat three to five times/leg.

Variation: Perform this exercise with knee bent on side to be stretched.

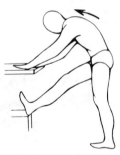

b

HAMSTRING STRETCH (STANDING)

1. Stand with leg to be stretched supported on a table or platform of comfortable height, knees straight.
2. Opposite foot should point straight ahead.
3. Slowly bend forward from hips until stretch is felt behind the knee of the leg on the table.
4. Hold 20 to 30 seconds. Repeat three to five times/leg.

HAMSTRING STRETCH (SITTING)

1. Sit on floor with leg to be stretched extended out in front of you.
2. Bend opposite leg and place sole of foot against knee of straight leg.
3. Slowly bend forward from hips toward foot of the straight leg until stretch is felt in back of knee.
4. Hold 20 to 30 seconds. Repeat three to five times/leg.

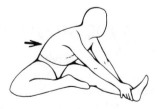

QUADRICEPS STRETCH

1. Stand close to a wall or chair for support, with the leg to be stretched extended behind you.
2. Hold foot of leg to be stretched with your hand, gently pulling the heel toward the buttock until a stretch is felt in the front of the thigh. Keep your hips stationary and gently extend your knee back.
3. Hold 20 to 30 seconds. Repeat three to five times/leg.

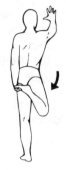

KNEES TO CHEST

1. Lie on back, with knees bent. Place hands behind knee.
2. Lift left knee, and with aid of arms, pull knee gently toward chest until stretch is felt in lower back.
3. Hold 20 to 30 seconds. Repeat three to five times/leg.

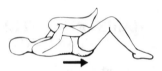

I-T BAND (STANDING)

1. Stand sideways, arm's length from wall, hand on wall for support, with leg to be stretched next to wall.
2. Slowly lean hip into wall until you feel a stretch along outside of hip.
3. Hold 20 to 30 seconds. Repeat three to five times/leg.

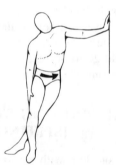

I-T BAND (SITTING)

1. Sit on the floor, with leg to be stretched crossed over opposite leg.
2. Pull leg in toward opposite shoulder until stretch is felt along outside of hip.
3. Hold 20 to 30 seconds. Repeat three to five times/leg.

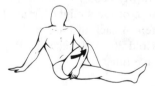

INNER THIGH

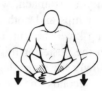

1. Sit on the floor, with knees bent and soles of feet against each other. This should not cause any knee pain.
2. Have your forearms give gentle stretching pressure against inner leg.
3. Hold 20 to 30 seconds. Repeat three to five times.

•LOWER EXTREMITY• STRENGTHENING PROGRAM

The knee is controlled by four muscle groups around the joint. These muscles can atrophy (waste away) very rapidly after an injury. Early in the rehabilitation of an injured knee or thigh, the following exercises are done mainly with the weight above the knee to reduce strain on the knee joint. As pain starts to subside after the first week, progress to exercises such as Patellar Program, Meniscus Knee Program, or Anterior Cruciate Knee Program.

STRAIGHT LEG RAISE-FLEXION

1. Lie face up on the floor.
2. Bend uninvolved knee and put foot on floor.
3. Slowly tighten the thigh muscle of the involved leg, performing a quad set.
4. Flex foot of involved leg toward nose.
5. Slowly lift entire leg 12 to 18 inches off floor.
6. Hold 3 seconds. Retighten the thigh muscle, and slowly lower to floor. Relax.
7. Perform ＿＿ sets, ＿＿ repetitions, ＿＿ times/day.

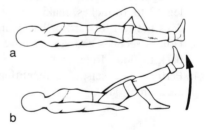

a

b

EXTENSION

1. Lie on your stomach, with a pillow under your hips and both legs straight.
2. Keeping knee straight, tighten the muscles in the posterior thigh and buttock, and slowly lift entire leg toward ceiling.
3. Hold 3 seconds and slowly lower leg. Relax.
4. Perform ____ sets, ____ repetitions, ____ times/day.

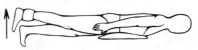

ADDUCTION

1. Lie on involved side, bending opposite leg and placing foot on floor behind involved leg.
2. Straighten involved knee, and slowly raise leg toward ceiling.
3. Hold 3 seconds and return leg to floor. Relax.
4. Perform ____ sets, ____ repetitions, ____ times/day.

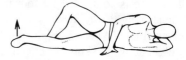

ABDUCTION

1. Lie on your side with involved leg up and bottom leg bent for balance.
2. Straighten involved knee and lift entire leg 12 to 18 inches, making sure hip does not roll forward or backward.
3. Hold 3 seconds and slowly lower leg back to floor. Relax.
4. Perform ____ sets, ____ repetitions, ____ times/day.

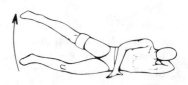

• PATELLAR PROGRAM •

Chondromalacia, more commonly known as runner's knee, is the term commonly used to describe several painful conditions of the knee related to the articulation between the patella (kneecap) and femur (thigh bone). This condition is not exclusive to runners but is associated with activities that involve repetitive bending of the knee. If possible, avoid squatting, excessive stair climbing, and kneeling during daily activities. Also avoid doing squats, leg presses, deep knee bends, and knee extensions on exercise equipment.

QUAD SETS

1. Lie face up on the floor.
2. Tighten the front thigh muscle (quadriceps) by attempting to push the back of your knee to the floor. Make the leg as stiff as possible.
3. Hold 5 seconds, relax 5 seconds.
4. Perform ____ sets, ____ repetitions, ____ times/day.

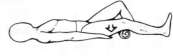

STRAIGHT LEG RAISE-FLEXION

1. Lie face up on the floor.
2. Bend uninvolved knee and put foot on floor.
3. Slowly tighten the thigh muscle of the involved leg, performing a quad set.
4. Flex foot of involved leg toward nose.
5. Slowly lift entire leg 12 to 18 inches off floor.
6. Hold 3 seconds. Retighten the thigh muscle and slowly lower to floor. Relax.
7. Perform ____ sets, ____ repetitions, ____ times/day.

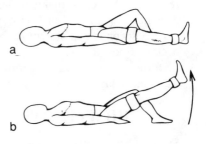

a

b

ADDUCTION

1. Lie on involved side, bending opposite leg and placing foot on floor behind involved leg.
2. Straighten involved knee and slowly raise leg toward ceiling.
3. Hold 3 seconds and return leg to floor. Relax.
4. Perform ___ sets, ___ repetitions, ___ times/day.

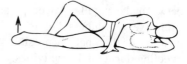

EXTENSION

1. Lie on your stomach, with a pillow under your hips and both legs straight.
2. Keeping knee straight, tighten the muscles in the posterior thigh and buttock, and slowly lift entire leg toward ceiling.
3. Hold 3 seconds and slowly lower leg. Relax.
4. Perform ___ sets, ___ repetitions, ___ times/day.

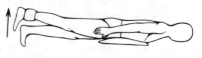

ABDUCTION

1. Lie on your side, with involved leg up and bottom leg bent for balance.
2. Straighten involved knee and lift entire leg 12 to 18 inches, making sure hip does not roll forward or backward.
3. Hold 3 seconds and slowly lower leg back to floor. Relax.
4. Perform ___ sets, ___ repetitions, ___ times/day.

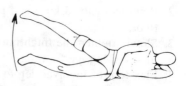

HIP FLEXION

1. Sit in a straight-backed chair, with feet on floor and knees bent.
2. Slowly raise involved knee toward ceiling.
3. Hold 3 seconds and slowly lower knee to starting position. Relax.
4. Perform ___ sets, ___ repetitions, ___ times/day.

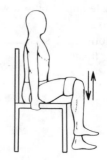

SHORT ARC QUADRICEPS

1. Lie face up on the floor with a small pillow or towel roll (6- to 8-inch diameter) under involved knee.

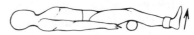

2. Slowly raise heel off floor by tightening knee.
3. Hold knee straight for 5 seconds.
4. Slowly lower heel to starting position.
5. Perform ____ sets, ____ repetitions, ____ times/day.

• MENISCUS KNEE PROGRAM •

This group of exercises is designed for those individuals who have suspected meniscus (cartilage) damage. The meniscus acts as a shock absorber between the joint surfaces of the tibia and femur. The meniscus can be torn or strained by twisting injuries. Excessive squatting and knee bending should be avoided in weight lifting. Avoid full arc knee extension against resistance when your knee is painful and/or swollen.

QUAD SETS

1. Lie face up on the floor.
2. Tighten the front thigh muscle (quadriceps) by attempting to push the back of your knee to the floor. Make the leg as stiff as possible.

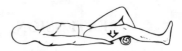

3. Hold 5 seconds, relax 5 seconds.
4. Perform ____ sets, ____ repetitions, ____ times/day.

STRAIGHT LEG
RAISE-FLEXION

1. Lie face up on the floor.
2. Bend uninvolved knee and put foot on floor.
3. Slowly tighten the thigh muscle of the involved leg, performing a quad set.
4. Flex foot of involved leg toward nose.
5. Slowly lift entire leg 12 to 18 inches off floor.
6. Hold 3 seconds. Retighten the thigh muscle and slowly lower to floor. Relax.
7. Perform ____ sets, ____ repetitions, ____ times/day.

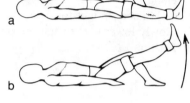
a
b

ADDUCTION

1. Lie on involved side, bending opposite leg and placing foot on floor behind involved leg.
2. Straighten involved knee and slowly raise leg toward ceiling.
3. Hold 3 seconds and return leg to floor. Relax.
4. Perform ____ sets, ____ repetitions, ____ times/day.

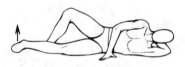

EXTENSION

1. Lie on your stomach, with a pillow under your hips and both legs straight.
2. Keeping knee straight, tighten the muscles in the posterior thigh and buttock, and slowly lift entire leg toward ceiling.
3. Hold 3 seconds and slowly lower leg. Relax.
4. Perform ____ sets, ____ repetitions, ____ times/day.

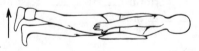

ABDUCTION

1. Lie on your side, with involved leg up and bottom leg bent for balance.
2. Straighten involved knee and lift entire leg 12 to 18 inches, making sure hip does not roll forward or backward.
3. Hold 3 seconds and slowly lower leg back to floor. Relax.
4. Perform ____ sets, ____ repetitions, ____ times/day.

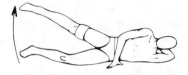

HAMSTRING CURLS

1. Lie on your stomach, with a pillow under your hips and both legs straight.
2. Slowly bend involved knee to 45- to 60-degree angle.
3. Hold 3 seconds and slowly lower the leg to starting position. Relax.
4. Perform ____ sets, ____ repetitions, ____ times/day.

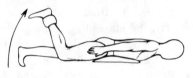

SHORT ARC QUADRICEPS

1. Lie face up on the floor, with a small pillow or towel roll (6- to 8-inch diameter) under involved knee.
2. Slowly raise heel off floor by tightening knee.
3. Hold knee straight for 5 seconds.
4. Slowly lower heel to starting position.
5. Perform ____ sets, ____ repetitions, ____ times/day.

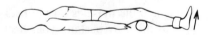

• ANTERIOR CRUCIATE KNEE PROGRAM •

This group of exercises is designed for those individuals who have ligamentous laxity in the knee, which is strongly suggestive of a stretched or torn anterior cruciate ligament. This problem is often caused by a hyperextension-type injury. As with all knee injuries, quadriceps development is important. With this particular problem hamstring strengthening to stabilize the joint is of special importance.

With an anterior cruciate deficient knee, it is to your advantage to have tighter than normal hamstrings. Light stretching before and after athletic activity is suggested. *Do not stretch aggressively.*

QUAD SETS

1. Lie face up on the floor.
2. Tighten the front thigh muscle (quadriceps) by attempting to push the back of your knee to the floor. Make the leg as stiff as possible.
3. Hold 5 seconds, relax 5 seconds.
4. Perform ____ sets, ____ repetitions, ____ times/day.

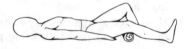

HAMSTRING SETS

1. Lie face up on the floor, with knee slightly bent.
2. Tighten the muscles on the back of your thigh by pushing your heel down against the floor.
3. Hold 5 seconds, relax and hold 5 seconds.
4. Perform ____ sets, ____ repetitions, ____ times/day.

STRAIGHT LEG
RAISE-FLEXION

1. Lie face up on the floor.
2. Bend uninvolved knee and put foot on floor.
3. Slowly tighten the thigh muscle of the involved leg, performing a quad set.
4. Flex foot of involved leg toward nose.
5. Slowly lift entire leg 12 to 18 inches off floor.
6. Hold 3 seconds. Retighten the thigh muscle and slowly lower to floor. Relax.
7. Perform ____ sets, ____ repetitions, ____ times/day.

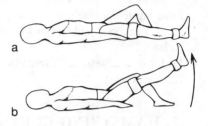

EXTENSION

1. Lie on your stomach, with a pillow under your hips and both legs straight.
2. Keeping knee straight, tighten the muscles in the posterior thigh and buttock, and slowly lift entire leg toward ceiling.
3. Hold 3 seconds and slowly lower leg. Relax.
4. Perform ____ sets, ____ repetitions, ____ times/day.

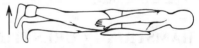

ABDUCTION

1. Lie on your side with involved leg up and bottom leg bent for balance.
2. Straighten involved knee and lift entire leg 12 to 18 inches, making sure hip does not roll forward or backward.
3. Hold 3 seconds and slowly lower leg back to floor. Relax.
4. Perform ____ sets, ____ repetitions, ____ times/day.

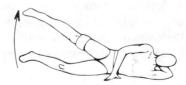

ADDUCTION

1. Lie on involved side, bending opposite leg and placing foot on floor behind involved leg.
2. Straighten involved knee, and slowly raise leg toward ceiling.
3. Hold 3 seconds and return leg to floor. Relax.
4. Perform ___ sets, ___ repetitions, ___ times/day.

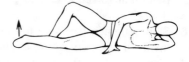

HAMSTRING CURLS

1. Lie on your stomach, with a pillow under your hips and both legs straight.
2. Slowly bend involved knee to 45- to 60-degree angle.
3. Hold 3 seconds and slowly lower the leg to starting position. Relax.
4. Perform ___ sets, ___ repetitions, ___ times/day.

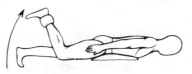

HAMSTRING CURLS (TUBING VARIATION)

1. Lie on your stomach as described above.
2. Attach tubing to ankle or shoe laces, and secure opposite end to non-moveable object (table leg, weight bench).
3. Slowly bend involved knee to 45- to 60-degree angle. Adjust tubing to give moderate to heavy resistance.
4. Hold 3 seconds and slowly lower the leg to starting position.
5. Perform ___ sets, ___ repetitions, ___ times/day.

Variation: Perform this advanced technique to emphasize power and endurance. Follow the instructions given, but adjust tubing to give mild resistance. Perform curl exercise at medium or high rate of speed until muscle fatigue is noted. Stretch hamstrings and repeat.

● ANKLE PROGRAM ●

Sprained ankle describes the condition of stretched or torn ligaments in your ankle. To prevent reinjury, you should perform the following strengthening and balance exercises as instructed by your therapist. Please let your therapist know if you have any questions or an increase in pain with the exercises.

RANGE OF MOTION

Plantar flexion

1. Move ankle as far as possible in a downward direction.
2. Perform ____ sets, ____ repetitions, ____ times/day.

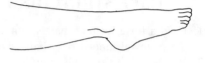

Dorsiflexion

1. Move ankle as far as possible in an upward direction.
2. Perform ____ sets, ____ repetitions, ____ times/day.

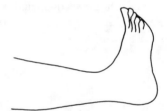

Inversion

1. Move ankle as far as possible in an inward direction.
2. Perform ____ sets, ____ repetitions, ____ times/day.

Eversion

1. Move ankle as far as possible in an outward direction.
2. Perform ＿＿ sets, ＿＿ repetitions, ＿＿ times/day.

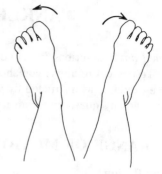

CALF STRETCHING

1. Hold a towel in both hands, with middle of towel looped over ball of foot.
2. Pull towel toward you, moving foot in an upward direction until stretch is felt in back of calf.
3. Hold 20 to 30 seconds and relax.
4. Perform ＿＿ sets, ＿＿ repetitions, ＿＿ times/day.

a

b

RESISTIVE EXERCISES WITH THERABAND

Plantar flexion

1. Place Theraband over ball of foot, holding one end of theraband in each hand.
2. Push foot in a downward direction, and slowly return to straight-up position.
3. Perform ＿＿ sets, ＿＿ repetitions, ＿＿ times/day.

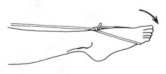

Dorsiflexion

1. Tie Theraband around table leg or other stationary object.
2. Loop Theraband over top of foot, and pull in an upward direction.
3. Slowly return to starting position.
4. Perform ____ sets, ____ repetitions, ____ times/day.

Inversion

1. Sit in a chair, with knee bent, Theraband tied to table leg.
2. Loop Theraband over foot, and pull in an inward direction.
3. Slowly return to starting position.
4. Perform ____ sets, ____ repetitions, ____ times/day.

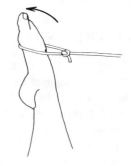

Eversion

1. Sit in a chair, with knee bent, Theraband tied to table leg.
2. Loop Theraband over foot, and pull in an outward direction.
3. Slowly return to starting position.
4. Perform ____ sets, ____ repetitions, ____ times/day.

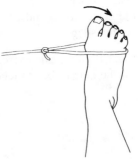

TOE RAISES

1. Stand with both feet on the floor.
2. Raise up on both toes, then slowly lower to feet-flat position.
3. Perform ____ sets, ____ repetitions, ____ times/day.
4. Progress to one foot.

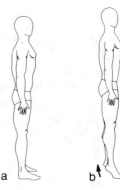

a   b

GASTROC-SOLEUS STRETCH

1. Stand at arm's length from a wall, palms flat against the wall, and the leg to be stretched straight behind you.
2. Bend opposite leg and place foot on the ground in front of you.
3. Keep heel of backward leg down, and keep arch up, toes curled under.
4. Slowly move your hips forward, keeping back straight until a stretch is felt in back of calf.
5. Hold 20 to 30 seconds. Repeat three to five times/leg.

Variation: Perform this exercise with knee bent on the side to be stretched.

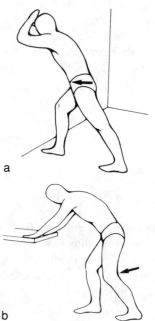

a

b

BALANCE EXERCISE

1. Practice standing on one leg with your eyes open.
2. When this is achieved with little or no difficulty for 1 minute, progress to standing on one leg with eyes shut.
3. This exercise will help to retrain your ankle's balancing ability.
4. Perform ____ times/day.

WINNING THE WEIGHTING GAME*
A lifestyle of eating for energy, health and weight control

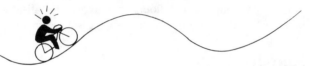

The Diet Cycle

Are you discouraged because no matter how you try to lose weight, it never works for very long? You either can't stay with whatever diet plan you're on; or you get too hungry; or you feel tired; or you get sick; or you feel deprived; or you lose the weight fast, then put it on again, **plus** some. The problem may be with the **way** you are trying to lose the weight: the "diet" plan you've chosen, your activity level, and your mental attitude. Let's look at some basic facts about weight, hunger, appetite, activity, and attitude.

Weight

First, there is NO magical cure or food or pill or "gimmick" that will make you lose weight effortlessly or permanently. The bottom line is still:

Note. From *Winning the Weighting Game*, 1984, Milwaukee, WI: Good Samaritan Medical Center. Copyright 1984 by Good Samaritan Medical Center. Reprinted by permission of Sinai Samaritan Medical Center.

CALORIES IN (FOOD) + CALORIES OUT (ACTIVITY) = WEIGHT CHANGE

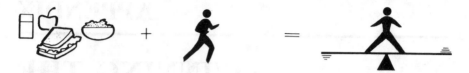

For health reasons, weight loss needs to be achieved gradually. When you try to lose weight too fast, more than 2-4 pounds per week, your body is tearing down vital organ and **muscle** tissue instead of fat. So make progress toward your weight loss goal "steady", not "fast".

Hunger and Appetite

Second, your body has some natural survival signals called hunger and appetite. If you try to ignore these signals (like going all day without eating), when you do finally give in to them you will eat more to satisfy your intense hunger. So it's better to eat in a way that keeps you from getting too hungry. Eat regularly throughout your waking hours and avoid the all-too-common pattern of no breakfast, little or no lunch, and a huge supper or binge eating in the evening.

Activity

No one can lose weight effectively—and KEEP it off—without changing his or her lifestyle to increase the activity level. Activity is the other side of the equation with food in changing weight. So . . . move it to lose it!

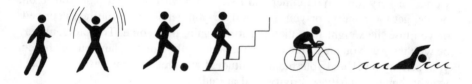

Attitude

Stop thinking: "DIET"!

Start thinking: "LIFESTYLE"!

No one can "diet" forever, because depriving yourself, physically or psychologically, leads to craving. What you **can** do is start making **choices** about the kinds of foods and how to prepare them for use on a day-to-day basis. In other words, instead of a "diet plan" that deprives you, think in terms of a "lifestyle"—of changing old habits that are causing you to gain weight, to new habits that become your way of life.

Height/Weight Guidelines*

(without shoes) Height	Low	(without clothes) Average	High
Women			
5 ft.	100	109	118
5 ft. 1 in.	104	112	121
5 ft. 2 in.	107	115	125
5 ft. 3 in.	110	118	128
5 ft. 4 in.	113	122	132
5 ft. 5 in.	116	125	135
5 ft. 6 in.	120	129	139
5 ft. 7 in.	123	132	142
5 ft. 8 in.	126	136	146
5 ft. 9 in.	130	140	151
5 ft. 10 in.	133	144	156
5 ft. 11 in.	137	148	161
6 ft.	141	152	166

(without shoes) Height	Low	(without clothes) Average	High
Men			
5 ft. 3 in.	118	129	141
5 ft. 4 in.	122	133	145
5 ft. 5 in.	126	137	149
5 ft. 6 in.	130	142	155
5 ft. 7 in.	134	147	161
5 ft. 8 in.	139	151	166
5 ft. 9 in.	143	155	170
5 ft. 10 in.	147	159	174
5 ft. 11 in.	150	163	178
6 ft.	154	167	183
6 ft. 1 in.	158	171	188
6 ft. 2 in.	162	175	192
6 ft. 3 in.	165	178	195

Source: U.S. Department of Agriculture

*These guidelines may underestimate desired body weight for athletic individuals, who have a greater amount of muscle tissue.

Food Facts

Just knowing where the calories are in foods does not insure a sound eating plan. Food Calories fall into 4 groups: fats, protein, carbohydrates (refined sugars and complex starches) and alcohol. Each type of food affects the body differently in appetite stimulation and satisfaction.

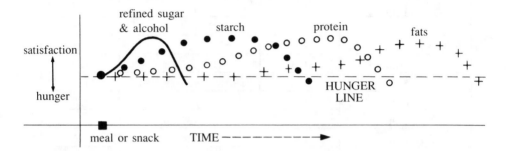

The types of calories you are eating will affect your hunger cycle. Refined sugars may immediately satisfy you, but leave you hungry again a short time later. Whereas starches, proteins and fats will satisfy you for a much longer period of time.

These four food calorie groups also provide different amounts of calories per weight (gram). Fats provide 9 calories per gram; proteins and carbohydrates provide 4 calories per gram; alcohol provides 7 calories per gram. Furthermore, fats, refined sugars and alcohol provide little or no nutrient value for the calories you get. Most foods combine two or more types of calories, but if you **reduce** your intake of those with a high amount of fat and refined sugar, and **increase** use of low fat proteins, complex starches and naturally occurring sugar in fruits, you can eat the same **amount** of food and insure balanced nutrition, but take in fewer calories!

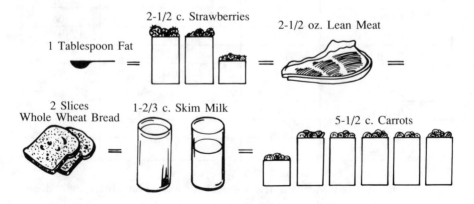

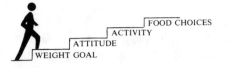

The Steps

1. Weight. Pick a reasonable goal—1-2 pounds per week (2-4 lbs/wk at the most). Losing weight too fast means intense hunger, muscle loss, low energy, and increased risk of infections and illness.

2. Attitude. Think POSITIVE—Think LIFESTYLE! Imagine the new, slimmer, healthier you! Think of the new **style** of life you will be living: one that will give you more energy, more satisfaction, less hunger and deprivation.

3. Activity. Activity does not have to mean a strenuous exercise program. Look for ways to increase activity in your daily schedule like parking an extra block from work and walking, taking the stairs instead of the elevator, getting off the bus a few blocks early and walking the rest of the way. *Warning—anyone over 35 yrs—or having a history of heart disease, high blood pressure or diabetes should consult a doctor before beginning an exercise program.

4. Food. The following general suggestions can be used in meal planning:

a. Limit use of refined sugars and fats wherever possible to reduce your intake of ''nutrient-empty'' calories.

b. Don't let yourself get too hungry. Eat at least 3 times per day—four to six is even better. Use fruits, vegetables and complex starches (without fat) as snacks.

c. Try using herbs and spices to flavor foods instead of salt to help reduce sodium intake. This is especially important for those with high blood pressure (hypertension).

d. Include a variety of foods from the protein, dairy, grain, fruit and vegetable groups to insure balanced nutrient intake.

How to . . .

Meal Planning.   First go through the various food categories and pick out those foods that you like and plan to use on a regular basis. If some of the foods on the "avoid" list are ones you are in the habit of using often, plan to prepare recipes without them, or find good substitutes. Plan for the meals and snacks that you will be eating on a weekly basis.

While your food selections should usually come from the moderate-to-low fat and sugar food lists, there may be times when foods on the AVOID list seem too hard to resist. Since restricting foods often leads to craving them, there are **positive** ways you can work these foods into your eating pattern. Your dietitian can show you how to either substitute them in your meal plan, or make positive decisions to use them on an occasional basis.

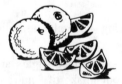

Your Kitchen.   Next, go through your kitchen and identify those foods that you will not be using, or will be trying to avoid. Can you do without them? Pick alternate foods from the list that you can use instead. For example, if you usually snack on bakery items in the afternoon, instead plan to use fresh fruit.

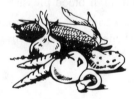

Shopping.   Now that you know which foods you want to use, and for which ones you need to find substitutes, write out a shopping list and USE it. Another tip: don't go to the store hungry! Plan to have a meal or snack at least 1/2 hour before shopping. If you are trying some new recipes, be sure to include the ingredients you don't have on hand on your shopping list.

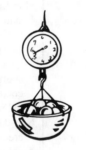

Food/Activity Records.   It's a good idea to keep a record of your food intake and activity pattern for the first several weeks. This can help you to identify problem times, so that you can change your patterns and avoid unconscious eating.

Portion Sizes.   No, you don't have to weigh your food forever. But it **is** important to measure out portions for a week or two until you have a good idea of how much you are really eating. You will need a scale and set of standard measuring cups and spoons. All measurements should be level. Also, if you eat slowly and give your stomach time to tell your brain that you are full (about 20 minutes), you will find you can eat less and still feel satisfied.

Foods to Avoid
High fat, sugar, cholesterol and/or low fiber

ANIMAL PROTEIN	DAIRY	VEGETABLE PROTEIN	VEGETABLES
Fatty beef, lamb, pork Spare ribs *Luncheon meat/ hot dogs Fried meats Liver, kidney Duck/goose *Sausage	*Whole milk cheese (cheddar, muenster, processed) Whole milk Sour cream, ice cream Cream cheese Cream, half & half Regular cottage cheese	*Salted & oil-processed nuts and seeds Peanut butter	Vegetables in cream or butter sauces Fried vegetables
FRUITS Fruits and juices with sugar/ syrup added	GRAINS/ STARCHES Cookies, pies, cakes Sweetened cereals Donuts *Snack crackers *Potato chips, corn chips Pancakes, waffles, biscuits	OTHERS Jams, jellies, syrups, sugar, honey, corn sweetener *Lard, bacon, salted pork, butter Hydrogenated vegetable shortening, coconut oil, palm oil Non-dairy creamers Alcohol Coconut Chocolate	

*High in Sodium

Foods to Use (Moderately)
Moderate fat, sugar, cholesterol and fiber

ANIMAL PROTEIN (Approximately 75 calories per portion listed)	DAIRY (Approximately 80 calories per portion listed)	VEGETABLE PROTEIN (Approximately 75 calories per portion listed)	VEGETABLE ("Free")
Lean beef, veal & pork: 1 ounce	*Lowfat cheese: 1 ounce (swiss, provolona, feta)	Raw or dry roasted nuts & seeds: 1 Tablespoon	*Canned vegetables & vegetable juices
Tuna in oil: scant 1/4 cup	Lowfat cottage cheese: 1/2 cup	Tofu: 3-1/2 ounces	*Sauerkraut, pickles
Poultry: 1 ounce	Lowfat (1%, 2%) milk: 3/4 cup		
Salmon, halibut, shrimp, lobster: 1 ounce or 1/4 cup	Fruited yogurts: 1/3 cup		
Eggs (3 per week): 1	Frozen yogurts: 1/3 cup		
*Ham, corned beef: 1 ounce	Sherbet: 1/3 cup		
Wild game: 1 ounce			
FRUITS (Approximately 60 calories per portion listed)	**GRAINS/ STARCHES** (Approximately 70 calories per portion listed)	**OTHERS** (Approximately 45 calories per portion listed)	
Canned fruit packed in juice or water: 3/4 cup	Refined, enriched breads & cereals, Refined pastas, White rice, Granolas: 1/2 cup	Added fats: salad dressings: 1 Tablespoon mayonnaise: 1 teaspoon margarine: 1 teaspoon	
Fruit juice: 1/2 cup	Cornbread: 1-1/2 inch cube	Avocados: 1/8	
Dried fruit: 1/4 cup	Bagels, English muffins: 1/2	Olives: 6	
Frozen fruit: 3/4 cup	Bialy: 1	Peanut & olive oil: 1 teaspoon	
	Graham crackers: 2 squares		
	Angel food cake, plain: 2" cube		
	Vanilla wafers: 5		
	*Pretzels: 25 sticks		

*High in Sodium

Food Group	Foods to Use Lowfat, sugar, cholesterol, higher fiber	Your Meal Plan Suggested servings for basic meal plan

ANIMAL PROTEIN
(Approximately 75
  calories per portion
  listed)
	Tuna in water: 1/3 cup
	Poultry (no skin): 1-1/2
	  ounces
	White fish—fresh fish:
	  1-1/2 ounces
	Egg white: 2
	Crab: 1/3 cup
	Low cholesterol egg
	  substitute: 1 serving
		(4-6 ounces)

DAIRY
(Approximately 80
  calories per portion
  listed)
	Part-skim mozzarella: 1
	  ounce
	Part-skim ricotta: 1/4 cup
	Skim milk: 1 cup
	  buttermilk: 1 cup
	Plain yogurt: 1/2 cup
	Parmesan cheese: 3-1/2
	  Tablespoons
		(2-4 servings)

VEGETABLE PROTEIN
(Approximately 75
  calories per portion
  listed)
	Dried beans & peas
	  (kidney, lima, soy
	  beans, lentils, split
	  peas, etc.): 1/3 cup
		(substitute for
		animal protein)

VEGETABLES ("Free")	Raw, fresh vegetables Fresh/frozen steamed vegetables	(as desired; minimum 2-4 servings per day)

FRUITS
(Approximately 60
  calories per portion
  listed)
	Raw, fresh fruit: 1
	  medium (1/2 banana)
		(3 servings)

GRAINS/STARCHES
(Approximately 70
  calories per portion
  listed)
	Shredded wheat: 3/4 cup
	Whole grain breads,
	  pastas & cereals: 1/2
	  cup
	Brown rice: 1/2 cup
	Bran cereals: 1/4 cup
	Potatoes, corn, peas, lima
	  beans, mixed
	  vegetables: 1/2 cup
	Popcorn (airpopped): 3
	  cups
		(5 servings)

OTHERS
(Approximately 45
  calories per portion
  listed)
	Vegetable oils: 1
	  teaspoon
		(1 teaspoon
		vegetable oil)
		(Total approximately
		1200 calories)

Sample Day's Meals
(For basic 1200 calorie meal plan)

Breakfast
1 c. skim/1% milk
3/4 c. cold cereal
1/2 c. orange juice
coffee/tea

Morning Snack
medium fresh fruit

Lunch
2-3 oz. lean meat/protein
1 slice whole wheat bread
lettuce/tomato slices
3/4 c. lowfat yogurt
1 c. strawberries

Afternoon Snack
5 whole wheat crackers
sugar-free soda

Supper
2-3 oz. lean meat/protein
medium baked potato
1 tsp. margarine
broccoli
tossed salad with diet dressing
sugar-free gelatin

Night Snack
3 c. popcorn (no added butter/margarine)
sugar-free lemonade

Free Foods

wine for cooking
natural flavoring extracts
natural seasonings (spices & herbs)
*low calorie salad dressing (less than 10 calories per serving)
unflavored or diet gelatin
coffee/tea, decaffeinated coffee, herbal tea
unsweetened lemonade
mint
sugar free sodas
sugar substitutes (in moderation)
vinegar
raw vegetables (in moderation)
*bouillon
*seasoning salts
*MSG (mono-sodium glutamate)
*meat tenderizers
*steak sauces
*soy sauce
*pickles
mustard, catsup (limit to 1 Tb./day)
sugarless gums

---

*High in Sodium

INDEX

ABOUT THE AUTHOR

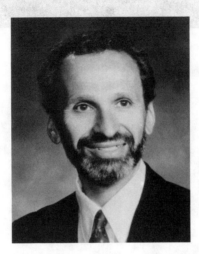

Gary N. Guten, MD, is an expert in the treatment of sports injuries. As medical director of the Sports Medicine Institute at Sinai Samaritan Medical Center in Milwaukee and an orthopedic surgeon, he treats hundreds of athletes every year. He also served for 10 years as the team physician for the Milwaukee Brewers. And as a marathon runner himself, Dr. Guten understands the pain and frustration of sports injuries.

In *Play Healthy, Stay Healthy*, Dr. Guten uses his experience to provide you with an easy-to-follow system for understanding your injuries and treating them in conjunction with your doctor.